Day-by-Day Gourmet

Braiden,

Much continued success.

[signature] '10

We are not human beings on a spiritual journey;
we are spiritual beings on a human journey.

TEILHARD DE CHARDIN

~ ~ ~

Make it your ambition to lead a quiet life:
You should mind your own business and work with your hands, . . .
so that your daily life may win the respect of outsiders.

1 THESSALONIANS 4:11–12a

Day-by-Day Gourmet

COOKBOOK

EAT BETTER · LIVE SMARTER · HELP OTHERS

GRAHAM KERR

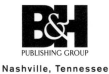

B&H
PUBLISHING GROUP

Nashville, Tennessee

ISBN: 978-0-8054-4488-9

Published by B & H Publishing Group,
Nashville, Tennessee

Dewey Decimal Classification: 613.2
Subject Headings: WEIGHT LOSS
                     NUTRITION
                     OBESITY

07 08 09 10 11   15 14 13 12 11 10 9 8 7 6 5 4 3 2 1

CONTENTS

· ·

AUTHOR'S NOTE

I've asked permission from the CEO of Day-by-Day Gourmet, Brad Voorhees, to use the name of his organization for this book's title.

In the interest of full disclosure (another way to say "walking in the light"), I need you to know that I am part of a team working with this innovative fledgling organization.

The Day-by-Day Gourmet customer assembly kitchens are currently quite small in number but may one day "alight" on a corner near you! Until that day it is my hope and indeed my prayer that the dishes and world-view issues raised in these pages will begin to edge your lifestyle choices toward both better health and a true celebration of our global table.

The abundant life that we have been promised as believers is one that is created to be shared with others—*a life lived so that everyone benefits!* When we began to turn toward this idea, we turned in the company of others who had themselves seen others turn.

Imagine, with us, only for a moment, what a glorious difference we could all make. Lives in which our previous harm would become resources that could bring healing to so many broken lives.

I believe, with all my heart, that the Day-by-Day Gourmet gathering kitchens can work side by side with this book. They can provide an extraordinary *occasional* service (see www.daybydaygourmet.com), and this book can go the second mile and help to provide that most desired of all gifts: ABUNDANT LIFE.*

*enough to share!

FOREWORD

Imagine a world where people have come to appreciate food in a way God, our Creator, has intended it to be. Food would be natural, free of any harmful additives and pollution as well as in total harmony and alignment with our body. People would consume the right foods in the right amounts, satisfying the bodies' needs to complete balance with the pleasures food should provide.

I truly believe that this is the world Graham and Treena Kerr have in mind when writing this book and have chosen it as their vision and mission. The reality of today obviously looks very different. People around the world have a most harmful relationship with food. In many countries obesity and other food-related health problems are rampant, while in other countries hunger and malnutrition takes a devastating toll on human lives. Hundreds of thousands of people are dying or fall seriously ill every year due to these travesties.

Graham and Treena are true pioneers in creating a passionate awareness of this problem and devote their energy to help people be restored to healthy relationships toward food. It is also a challenge to the food industry to be more responsible in the way they serve people.

In this book Graham takes a reader through a candid, insightful, and very personal revelation of his and Treena's journey from the most celebrated culinary celebrity, with a very hedonistic approach to food, to the humbling experience of being confronted by God and making a complete turnaround—they followed His call to become passionate and caring pioneers of a new healthy God-ordained philosophy of food with a new mission.

This book also provides the reader with simple tools to establish a wholesome lifestyle. It is also filled with many tasty and easy-to-make recipes from across the globe.

I personally thank God every day that He brought Graham and Treena into my life. My family and I have learned so much from them and have become keenly aware of the responsibility we as food professionals and leaders have to change the course in our world as it relates to food. They have also personally touched me in many ways, and I am truly honored and proud to call them friends.

Karl J. Guggenmos, MBA, AAC
Certified German Master Chef
University Dean of Culinary Education
Johnson & Wales University

PREFACE

To assess the progress of civilization in our world today is quite possibly beyond any one person, and to suggest an ability to do so would be extraordinary vanity.

I make no such claim, and yet I must set forth my concern about *one element of civilization*: our excess consumption of food while others suffer and die from insufficiency.

For a nation or nations to pursue such excess and be unwilling to include those left out of the essential, consistent distribution of food is, in my opinion, uncivilized behavior.

So where are we, as "developed" nations, in our cultural, social willingness to share out of our apparent abundance?

I could use all the measurements that others, better equipped than I, have already used and would simply echo their findings that *numerically* we are eating our abundance at the expense of our own health (and self-worth). Our overconsumption has not contributed to our pursuit of happiness; in fact, the opposite is often true!

And yet, in response to the pressure of our highly competitive food industry, we continue to make choices that lead to significant increases in overweight, obesity, and chronic diseases, which in turn contribute to ever escalating health-care costs.

Add it all up, and we are obviously in the midst of a mess of our own making!

~ ~ ~

There is an answer to our dilemma, and it begins with love—because God has commanded and God has promised. Therefore we love Him with *all* our heart, with *all* our soul, with *all* our mind, and we love our neighbor and *ourselves* with the same kind of love because in a loving *God we trust.*

It really doesn't matter if we are sick and want to be well, if we are well and don't want to be sick, or if we are caring for a loved one in either category. What comes first is our attitude, the way we see the world around us—as created, as a gift, as a responsibility and, most of all, as a celebration. Are we willing to simplify, encourage, and celebrate?

We celebrate our creative God and His wondrous works, which includes you, me, and all those we love.

Since what we consume and how we move about is a vital part of being well and having the *physical* part of our abundant life, then both cooking and movement can be seen as a valuable part of the Christian life.

It is in the way we blend the spiritual with the physical. The more seamless, the more resolve we can bring to our search for our very own lifestyle for a lifetime.

Our solution is obvious: "eat less and share more." We call this *outdulgence,* which is really a simple day-by-day *choice.* Do I consume a food or beverage in a volume (portion size) that *could* harm me? If so, then will I *choose* a smaller portion (that costs less) and avoid the personal harm and accumulate the monetary savings in order to provide for the needs of someone in a hopeless situation? What would have been indulgence now becomes outdulgence!

Christians are mandated by the most basic tenants of our faith to share in love with those in need, and many of us do share—*in part.* I believe that it's now time for another level of contribution that is entirely individual in nature.

We must ask ourselves: What are *my* personal measurements of consumption, and are they contributing to my health and the *protection* of the fruit of the spirit (love, joy, peace, patience, goodness, kindness, faithfulness, gentleness, self-control) in my life?

If there is *any* doubt, then we must be willing to prayerfully assess *our* personal behavior (see pp. 236/248) and its cost to both our health and the resources we could commit to another's life.

Individually this *solution* may seem insignificant when we consider what a government could do with our *tiny* tax contribution. However, if we did it through our churches and encouraged others in our churches to do the same, then we could lift up a new standard of social and cultural norms better suited to an apparently Christian nation.

Go out, go out through the gates;
prepare a way for the people!
Build it up, build up the highway;
clear away the stones!
Raise a banner for the peoples.
                              Isaiah 62:10

Let that banner be one of love, one that carries not one word of criticism or judgment of others. Our world lacks no critics; what we need is more contributors to the common good.

Graham Kerr
Mt. Vernon, Washington

My Pantry of Purpose-filled People

Acknowledgments

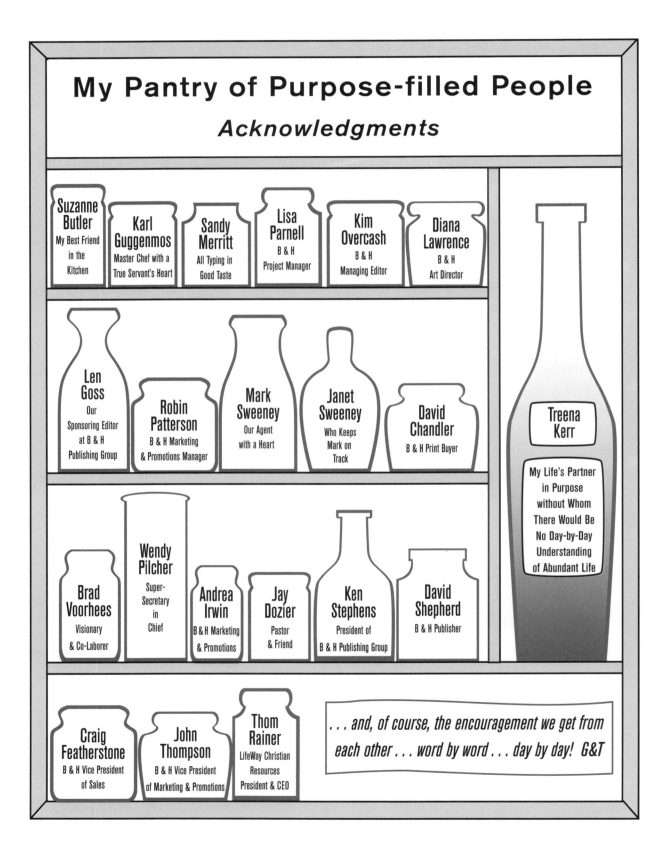

Suzanne Butler — My Best Friend in the Kitchen

Karl Guggenmos — Master Chef with a True Servant's Heart

Sandy Merritt — All Typing in Good Taste

Lisa Parnell — B & H Project Manager

Kim Overcash — B & H Managing Editor

Diana Lawrence — B & H Art Director

Len Goss — Our Sponsoring Editor at B & H Publishing Group

Robin Patterson — B & H Marketing & Promotions Manager

Mark Sweeney — Our Agent with a Heart

Janet Sweeney — Who Keeps Mark on Track

David Chandler — B & H Print Buyer

Treena Kerr — My Life's Partner in Purpose without Whom There Would Be No Day-by-Day Understanding of Abundant Life

Brad Voorhees — Visionary & Co-Laborer

Wendy Pilcher — Super-Secretary in Chief

Andrea Irwin — B & H Marketing & Promotions

Jay Dozier — Pastor & Friend

Ken Stephens — President of B & H Publishing Group

David Shepherd — B & H Publisher

Craig Featherstone — B & H Vice President of Sales

John Thompson — B & H Vice President of Marketing & Promotions

Thom Rainer — LifeWay Christian Resources President & CEO

. . . and, of course, the encouragement we get from each other . . . word by word . . . day by day! G&T

INTRODUCTION

Most cookbooks have a very small opening chapter and then cut to the chase with a selection of recipes. In our case, I've gone to some length to explain why we do what we do.

The danger with any prescribed food style is that when it is somehow connected to our inner spiritual life it can become a legalism—"If I eat this way then I'm a good person" or "If I eat this or that food, I'm a bad person." Nothing could be further from the truth!

Consider what Scripture says in Colossians 2: "Therefore don't let anyone judge you in regard to food and drink" (v. 16). "Let no one disqualify you, insisting on ascetic practices" (v. 18). "If you died with Christ to the elemental forces of this world why do you live as if you still belonged to the world? Why do you submit to regulations 'Don't handle, don't taste, don't touch?' All these regulations refer to what is destroyed by being used up; they are human commands and doctrines. Although these have the reputation of wisdom by promoting ascetic practices, humility and severe treatment of the body, they are not of any value against fleshly indulgence" (vv. 20–23).

In other words, you can't rely upon radical restrictive diets to deal with an inner conflict between your flesh and your spirit.

My entire message is that the only way to live with relative health in these extraordinary days is to let the fundamental principles of the kingdom of God, as expressed and lived by Jesus Christ, become the foundation for a *whole lifestyle.*

In our book *Recipe for Life* we discussed *whole lifestyle* as being represented by a needle. A needle on its own can be used to prick people, to needle them with pointed criticism. But when you pass your faith through the eye of the needle, it becomes an instrument of reconciliation, bringing two sides of something together to mend or to heal.

Jesus used His whole life to heal and to mend, to reconcile mankind to God. As Christ-followers, we should do no less!

In this book, therefore, we look at one aspect of our daily lifestyle—the way we eat and drink—and we ask ourselves, "What happens when I thread the 'eye' of my food lifestyle with my faith?" Can I *see* that overeating can cost more money, and that if I ate less I could save enough to help someone in desperate need? Can I *see* that by reducing my portion sizes I am benefiting my own life, reducing weight and the risk of diabetes and heart disease?

I submit that this lifestyle is *not* one of promoting ascetic practices, humility, or severe treatment of the body with strict dietary rules. I do believe that it *is* a *way of escape* from the cultural lifestyle that is presently overwhelming our lives.

"No temptation has overtaken you except what is common to humanity. God is faithful and He will not allow you to be tempted beyond what you are able, but with the temptation He will also provide a way of escape, so that you are able to bear it" (1 Cor. 10:13).

God truly loves us enough to have us understand that there are *treats,* and that He loves to see our joy as we delight in the taste, aroma, color, and texture of a food. I also believe that it grieves Him when we go beyond the *treat* and expose ourselves to the *threat* that almost always comes from today's unreasonable portions.

Treena and I don't see our lifestyle choices as a legalism but rather as a *spring-board.* We bounce up and down on an idea (or a recipe) to get the feel of it. Then we do our own dive into the waters of our circumstance.

And that is exactly what we want for you. We want you to fashion your own dive because you alone understand the waters of your unique circumstances. All you need to do is to bounce up and down on our "springboard" ideas to get the feel of them and then decide how you might turn your dive into a lifestyle for a lifetime.

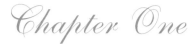

MY NEW WORLDVIEW

It seems to me that we are living in a pivotal time—for our nations and our world.

If we can learn how to share out of our relative abundance with those in need, we may well survive. If we cannot—or will not—then clearly our days may be numbered.

I have lived long enough to have had two worldviews. In the first, I wanted the world to see me; in the second, I wanted to see the world and meet its needs—or at least a few of them.

In the first, until I was forty, I succeeded on the outside and failed on the inside. In the second, I've become, for some, vaguely suspect in my apparent motives. Yet I'm alive inside and filled with hope for a better future.

This book is a good example of this change in worldviews—from indulgence to *outdulgence,* which my wife, Treena, and I see as a major source of hope for all mankind.

What individuals consume and properly digest on a regular basis has an enormous effect upon who we are. It isn't just about being sick and being well, or about being heavy or light; it's really about how much we consume and how much we choose to share. There are appropriate balancing points for every one of us.

I have cooked for myself and my family for as long as I have been able to safely reach

a stove top. My best known occupation was when I tried to understand how the peoples of this world cooked and ate and then passed that information on through television as the Galloping Gourmet.

I *galloped* because we did 195 shows a year and did our research in the nations from which the dishes came. We girdled the world twenty-eight times in our search, and *gallop* therefore was a perfect description. *Gourmet* has always been a commercial word to describe a proper marriage between wine and food. By proper, I mean sensually balanced so as to become an integrated delight—or pleasure.

Our program, which Treena produced and co-created with me, was, in its time, an enormous success in many nations. We had our humble beginnings in New Zealand when there were only fifty TV sets in the whole nation. That's when I had a 100 rating!

All my early food fumblings were accepted because I was the only game in town. When Australia beckoned, I learned the meaning of competition and survival. I was desperate to survive and fought like a drowning man going down for the third time in seas of self-doubt.

Who was I to deserve a viewer's attention; what *did* I really know? It was never enough to add up to a glimmer of self-worth.

3

When the United States media called, our world speeded up, and millions watched as I leapt my episodes like hurdles in a race for the finish.

We were in the midst of abundance, savoring the very best, watched and to some extent idolized, and yet we had no time to reflect on values, or community, or even the short-term future of our own family. All that seemed to matter was to jump another episodic hurdle and get set up for the next.

It was then that, with so little energy left, we were hit from behind by a vegetable truck. Our injuries brought the program to a dead stop in the spring of 1971. Treena's trauma led all the way to a lung resection, and I had a partial paralysis of one side.

We did try to fulfill our obligations, but leaping over chairs with a wine glass and cavorting in general was beyond me. And without Treena there was no joy in the journey.

We went off in search of healing along with our previously neglected children— Tessa, our English firstborn; Andy, our New Zealand middle son; and Kareena, our Australian. If we had had a child in Canada, the Queen might have given us a commonwealth medal!

We sailed some twenty-four thousand miles in our search, and we did get better—at least physically. Inside, however, we carried all the pain and despair caused by competition without apparent purpose other than survival.

We were still drowning, and now was the summer of our discontent! I had come as far as I could go, and there was no end in sight;

nothing of any value beckoned. It seemed to us that we had now been there and done that—and so what?

Upon our return to dry land with a new, much healthier way of eating but without a new way of living, we settled down to eat and yet be eaten by a profound sense of failure. Treena especially plunged into a deep well of depression, and I watched, unable to provide a solution no matter how hard I tried.

Our salvation came through our maid, Ruthie Turner. Ruthie wasn't a *real* maid. She was, in fact, a *real* missionary (in her heart) who simply wanted to get to Haiti to serve her hurting brother and sisters.

She began by earning our respect through the works of her hands. She did a great job on our 10,800 square-foot home.

She followed this with a prayer vigil along with her inner city Pentecostal Holiness Church in Wilmington, Delaware.

Eventually, after several months, she was bold enough to say to Treena, "Mrs. Kerr, why don't you give your troubles to God." Treena replied, "Alright, God, if You are so clever, You deal with me because I can't."

(I always like Treena to tell you what happened next; it is, after all, the most intimate of all personal stories, the day when everything started to become new. She describes it all in our first book that we coauthored, *Recipe for Life*.)

~ ~ ~

Throughout it all, I had the most wonderful of all spiritual opportunities—I was left alone to observe a genuine miracle. Scripture talks about coming out of darkness into God's wonderful light. Well, Treena had stepped over, and the difference really was night and day. Treena changed *utterly* and literally overnight.

She didn't have to *say* anything; all she did was live out her new life amongst all her family who knew her so well. Within a few months, every one of us believed, and we were all hungry for our own personal relationship. I've written about my own search along with Treena in the prequel to this book called *Recipe for Life,* largely because for me the transition was to take more time. There was so much self-indulgence to unwind.

My story is largely about appearance, approval, and financial security. All these preoccupations gradually diminished and in time reversed, but that, as they say, is the other story. For now, in this book, my purpose is to record how my coming to faith literally invaded my proficiency.

So . . . what does happen when a gourmet meets his God?

At the high point of my gourmet career, I had earned the "Broken Wooden Spoon Award" from Weight Watchers. They actually sent me a spoon snapped in two along with a letter to explain that, in their opinion, I was the "most dangerous man in the world" (to those wanting to lose weight).

The mass media dubbed me "The High Priest of Hedonism" and, borrowed from the show's galloping title, they spun the term "Hedonist in a Hurry." I looked it up to be certain and found that a hedonist's chief end (and virtue) in life was to pursue pleasure.

The cap appeared to fit, so I wore it—with gusto!

The suggestions that I might be doing someone harm came occasionally, but since they got in the way of my survival, I treated them with lighthearted scorn. I had chosen how I would live my life; so others were perfectly free to choose theirs—only just get out of my way because at least I was a success.

In ancient Greece, a writer philosopher posed an interesting question in his work: "Which man does the greater good to man— the one that makes you laugh or the one who makes you weep?"

I made people laugh, and that, along with our bank account, was all the feedback I needed.

~ ~ ~

Food is an extraordinarily powerful temptation. To live we must eat; we simply cannot "give it up."

Food is judged by *all* the senses—by sight, taste, texture (touch), smell, and even hearing (sizzle?). When all the senses are pleased, there is a great desire to repeat the sensation and perhaps look for larger and larger portions.

Cooks from the beginning of recorded culinary history in both China and India have known how salt, sweet, sour, and bitter can be juggled together to create truly addictive sensations. We have now reached a degree of sophistication (definition: "to make false") in recipe development when addictive levels of salt, fats, and sugars have been served up in enormous portions simply in order to gain or retain a share of today's consumer market.

Content and size is not caused by consumer demand. Today's temptations, inflated as they often are, have their roots not in commercial greed, but in sheer survival. Today's "food entrepreneurs" and blue chip manufacturers are strongly motivated by enormous competitive pressure and are assisted by the most agile advertising and promotion industry that the world has ever seen.

Every day we, modern consumers, are urged to buy into some form of excess consumption, and we are promised that we will enjoy it and come back for more. By and large these promises are prophetic; we do return, we do eat more and more, *and* we are now suffering from self-inflicted wounds.

Scripture speaks of there being no temptation given to man other than that which is normal, and even then God has given us a way to stand up under that temptation (see 1 Cor. 10:13).

Even the Lord's Prayer has us cry out to the Father: "Give us this day our daily bread . . . lead us not into temptation . . . deliver us from evil."

My very strongly held opinion is that the only message able to help us to stand up under the modern food marketing system is the gospel of Jesus Christ.

The Great Commandment really says it all: "Love the Lord your God with all your heart, with all your soul, and with all your mind. This is the greatest and most important commandment. The second is like it: Love your neighbor as yourself. All the Law and the Prophets depend on these two commandments" (Matt. 22:37–40).

This wasn't a suggestion—this was a commandment that embraced *all* the law and *all* the prophets.

So, what is our response as we now live out our generation (generally, twenty years) in the gospel—the one hundred and first generation to receive the baton passed on to us by faithful men and women of God?

We can love God for everything He has done and continues to do for us, and in the same spirit (without criticism or condemnation of anyone) we can lovingly share out of our abundance with our neighbors in need.

This then is my new worldview. What I used to consume and actively encourage others to consume has been gradually transformed until, today, what used to harm us has now been converted into both time and money that can heal others—and ourselves.

Let me try to illustrate this change with a simple idea. We call it . . .

Chapter Two

THE TALE OF TWO COOKIES

· ·

I doubt you will ever find a better example of obsessive compulsive behavior than the one I'm about to confess. I'd like you to know that I don't make this manifestation a regular part of my lifestyle. It was only, as they say, a test!

I decided to count how many cookies I ate each day. I kept a tally with both dates and times for a month! I did this for a purpose, wanting to see who, in our home, was responsible for the ever shrinking supply.

It was I!

On a good (or was it bad) day, I'd munch my way through five, sometimes six. My average was four.

Now please notice I haven't asked you to count yours. I don't want to make comparisons with anybody–*ever!*

"Comparisons" my father used to say, "are always odious." Not only odious, but they lead, inevitably so it seems, to criticism and even judgment of others, and this, I've found out, is not only disobedient but also deadly!

I went a stage further with my cookie investigation and found that the commercially baked cookies averaged 100 calories each at a cost of 17 cents. I did the math on my averages over one month. Thirty times 100 calories was 3,000–or for one year, 36,000–and that was for only one. For four cookies, I totaled 144,000 calories.

My subcutaneous fatty tissue (the bulg-

ing on my waist) adds up to 3,500 calories for each pound. So I divided my 144,000 intake of calories by 3,500 and was shocked to see that what I ate added up to the calories needed to provide for forty pounds of fatty bulge, with no added nutritional benefit!

But that wasn't the end of it. What about the cost?

My store-bought cookies (I don't make cookies at home for what, by now, must be pretty obvious reasons) cost 17 cents each. Once again I multiplied 1,440 cookies by 17 cents and arrived at $244.80 and that was just for me!

Knowing that the loss of only ten pounds would get me out of the overweight classification, as outlined in the "Body Mass Index." (I was a 24, which made me *just* overweight. See p. 245 for a chart to measure your BMI).

Lose ten pounds and I'd be normal–imagine being *normal* at last, something I'd tried for half my life to be anything but!

Treena decided to join me in my quest for normality and never to exceed two cookies a day. Between the two of us, we would save about $244.50 and possibly lose up to ten pounds–even in our imperfect world.

The money came out of our food budget. It would have obviously been swallowed up in some other minor expenditure that we would never had noticed had we not, on the first day of each month, deducted our $10.20 from the food budget and transferred it to a new savings account called Outdulgence.

We let this little sum gradually increase as we added other changes, some major, others minor. Before long, we had easily exceeded the six-hundred-dollar-a-year mark. We had begun praying to see where we would best send our "savings" since it was really *new* money and beyond our normal tithe commitment to our church.

We made our first compassionate connections (out of lifestyle changes) with Compassion International. We did so because we had carefully researched their operation and found it exemplary (and still do after more than twelve years).

In the midst of this style of giving, we had the additional idea that we should commit to give for three-year periods. This would give our old habits a good chance to die out and those we supported a solid period of reliable support, avoiding the constant problem we call "fickle-funding."

It is a fact of life, regrettably, that Christian ministries must compete with modern marketing for their donors' disposable income. Over the years, this has led some to adopt secular fund-raising techniques for Kingdom purposes. In turn, it has led to both cynicism and resistance, even to judgment, and as a result of all three, an unreliable source of income for ministries that want to declare the faithfulness of a God who loves in so many practical ways—until the trickle becomes fickle and dries up.

To our three-year commitment (the period of Jesus' full-time earthly service) we added a written promise: "If we choose to move on, we will give you, at the end of year two, a full year's notice *and* we promise to give you our reason for change so that you may consider the issue and alter some practice (if possible) to allow our continuance."

This has worked so well that we have converted it to an EFT service (Electronic Fund Transfer) in our local church, where we add 10 percent to each monthly gift to cover the administrative overhead.

Now, you may ask, has this resulted in others doing the same?

It did, some years back in a previous church, but not, we regret, in another one we attended for several years.

Regret? Well, not really! Looking back over our prayer notes, we can see that our role (Treena's and mine) is to hold hands, as we did when we met at school, laugh and skip and let "seeds" pour out of our pockets as we go—like two innocent Johnny Appleseeds—simply letting the idea of outdulgence *go!*

We don't plant or tend or prune or harvest. Our job is to sew and therefore never to regret. If the seed grows in your heart, we will eventually be overjoyed when all becomes known.

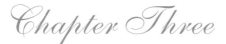

TREAT OR THREAT?

As we have shared, my cookie consumption amounted to 144,000 calories with no added nutrients except for the energy—or if you prefer, 144,000 "empty" calories.

Does that mean that cookies must now be viewed as somehow *evil*? I don't think so. In fact, I'm sure they are not, at least when consumed in reason.

The famed pharmacologist Paracelcius once said, "All things are toxic; it's just a matter of the dose."

Perhaps we can agree that excess consumption of a toxic substance that can kill you is not appropriate human behavior and not a godly attribute.

So could excess (in and of itself) be evil, especially if it is the direct cause of harm?

A war or primitive injustice can cause harmful *under*consumption, leading to disease and often death. Is *that* evil? I think so.

So what is the difference if the end result is the same?

Privation or excess can both be deadly. The cause and effect could therefore share the same source—evil.

My problem was to try to sort out what constituted *excess*. Obviously, this would change individual by individual according to their weight, health, and possibly their genetic predisposition to certain diseases inherited from their parents.

Previously I suggested that "there is an appropriate *balancing point* for every one of us," a point at which we stop consuming and start sharing.

Where we *individually* put that balancing point will, to some extent, advance or destroy what we know today as civilization.

It seems obvious, at least to me, that to continue to knowingly consume excess to our own harm when we are acutely aware of at least thirty thousand children dying every single day is actually uncivilized behavior.

So, how do we find our balancing point? And there's the rub; it isn't an exact science because we don't eat or behave in a rigid measurable way day after day.

All we can do is take a stab at finding it—by doing something like I did.

I was born with a tiny gap in my brain. (Treena likes to say that the hole is between my left and right ear!) The problem with this seven-millimeter hole is that tiny blood vessels find it and "curl up" in the space, only to rupture if my blood pressure goes through the roof, as it has on two spectacular occasions.

I have been told to keep my blood pressure below 130/80. If I can't I will have to be medicated.

Since I take no medication, not even a multivitamin, I chose to lose about twelve pounds and stop being overstressed ("Be anxious for nothing" [Phil. 4:6 NKJV]).

It appears to have worked.

We lose weight by reducing the consumption of empty calories, highly concentrated animal fats, or refined starchy carbohydrates and also by increasing the way we move, subsequently burning calories as energy. Put simply, eat less and move more and you lose weight.

In my case, the *eat less* came from the foods that did me the most predictable harm. I reduced my meat from 8 to 10 ounces per day to 4 ounces and cookies from 4 to 2. I removed chocolate for more than 20 years and now eat 1 ounce very occasionally. I use less sodium. I've halved the amount of bread by keeping to a whole multigrain organic "artisan" bread; it is so satisfying that a second slice is unnecessary.

I could go on and on—*in fact, I do.* In every single recipe in this book I've reduced portion sizes to what I call R/M for "reasonable/moderate."

Now I grant you, my portions won't *immediately* please a red-blooded American male, but they may save his life downstream.

Whatever you choose to do, I urge you to be obsessive compulsive for just one week! Make a careful note of any small issue in your lifestyle that you *think* just might be causing harm to either yourself or those you love. (For an assessment listing, see Favorite Foods charts starting on p. 236.)

Keep track of it, use your supermarket receipts to capture and average the cost, *imagine* what you could do to consume less, and then actually save some money!

It helps if the whole family agrees to the change (or changes) and fully participates in finding your compassionate connection. Perhaps, as we have done, a child somewhere might never had known life were it not for your family's "sacrifice."

It has helped Treena and me to recognize that in our sacrifice, we actually converted a possible *threat* (four cookies) to a *treat* (two cookies). The only difference in those words, since they both end in eat is the letter H, and that, my friends, stands for *high* in volume and repetition. If you cut out the H factor, you discover another H— healing both for yourself and others. That's the essence of outdulgence.

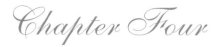

Chapter Four

OBSESSION OR SURVIVAL?

The underlying promise of a modern democracy is freedom. We have the freedom to speak our minds, to gather together to express our opinions, and even to seek another government if we choose. We are subject to laws written with the common good at heart. After that? Why, we are on our own, with our conscience as our guide.

This is where, as Christians, we enter the realm of the moral law, which, for the most part, forms the foundation of the law of the land and then ventures on to be "written on our hearts."

Somewhere on the roadway from common law to moral law it sometimes gets foggy. The road conditions are controlled by a continuous array of "billboarded" advertisements. The idea behind those billboards is to remind us of both our needs and our wants, and then to *sell* us something.

One recent roadside display asked a question: "Is your stomach stuck on empty?" It then went on to propose "At exit 320, fill 'er up with friendly food. It's highway heaven!"

Notice that the message was pitched to a possible *need*—we are hungry. It goes on to promise a bellyful, a smile, and a pleasant experience.

I remembered it because, after several hundred miles of driving, it was a relief from the standard "All you can eat!"

Once again, grab the attention by connecting to a possible need and then follow with an attractive promise.

This may net you one customer, but how do you get that impulse purchaser to become a "franchised" regular until the volume reaches upward toward the "golden arches" and their $38 billion a year turnover (the same amount, within a billion or so, that U.S. citizens spend annually trying to lose weight!).

All of this to say that the only way Treena and I have managed to stand up under these multiple temptations is to become borderline obsessive compulsive. We keep journals and charts and complete them every single day of our lives. We get up early enough to have a "quiet time," about one hour, and during that time we jot down what we ate the previous day (while it's still warm in our memories).

Now comes the hard part (when the obsessions border on compulsion): we weigh ourselves, take our blood pressure on a simple wrist cuff, and Treena records her fasting blood glucose on a small meter called a One Touch™. We both carry a pedometer to measure the distance we walk each day in steps, and I work out how many servings of fruit and vegetables we ate. When we are on the road, we add the altitude because it affects her blood sugars.

All of this adds up to less than fifteen minutes of compulsion (or is it obsession?). We then get on with our daily devotions.

The late and very great Julia Child was fond of saying, "You can eat anything if you eat it in moderation." To which I would counter, "Yes, Julia, we all agree, but how do you *measure* what is moderate?"

The only way I know how to do that is to keep a record. Then I have a cause and an effect—both Treena and I can see when we've exceeded our feed limit. It's there in black and white!

We now have almost ten years of monthly charts (see example layout on pp. 246–47) and can see the benefit to our weight and overall health our decisions have made since 1987. This record is also of enormous value to our medical friends who keep a loving and caring eye on Treena's progress.

I have gained *my* benefit by having so far avoided the necessity to take any medications or supplements, and Treena put off the need for a bypass operation for 19 years.

This would be enough were our personal well-being a strong enough motive to make wise choices. But . . .

It isn't and never has been!

Psychology 101 states flatly that if man is left alone (without external influence) he will always pursue pleasure and avoid pain.

The excess consumption of food and drink is momentary *pleasure.* That's how we get *instant gratification.* The long-term impact of excess is disease and pain. The problem lies in the extended gap between the pleasure and the pain.

When the flesh fights with the spirit, the flesh tends to win, especially when aggressively encouraged by advertising. This is why we need to venture further toward the moral law, and here we find some excellent biblical guidance for the Christian: "If you have died with Christ to the elementary principals of the world [Psychology 101 and billboards], why, as if you were living in the world, do you submit yourself to decrees such as 'Do not handle, do not taste, do not touch!' (which refer to things destined to perish with use)—in accordance with the commandments and teachings of men? These are matters which have, to be sure, the appearance of wisdom in self-made religion and self-abasement and severe treatment of the body, but are of no value against fleshly indulgence" (Col. 2:20–23 NASB).

These verses spoke to me about every kind of diet ever invented: high fat, low fat, low carb, . . . you name it. It's all about suggesting that something or things are bad for you. If you cut them out—bingo, you lose weight and feel *wonderful* about yourself.

After a few weeks or months, however, you've nibbled your way back up the scales and feel *awful* about yourself. Keep this up for long and your life is a *yo-yo,* with self firmly fixed in the crosshairs of your own obsession.

If self-control can't deal with fleshly indulgence (sponsored by a world full of billboards), then what can?

Outdulgence can! Keep a daily record, find a compassionate connection, and turn your flesh into "fruit." This really is your double benefit, and it's powerful enough to help you *to stand.*

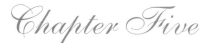

ADDICTION AND THE WAY BACK

Once again, I'd like to return to that balancing point between treat and threat, that place where we stop consuming and start to share.

What happens when we move over that point and become so attached to something that it simply takes over.

I've known what this feels like. I had been exposed to multiple temptations and knew enough, now and again, to want to back out. It was always "when I get to the end of this pack of cigarettes or this bottle of Chateau Margaux or this bar of Cadbury's Fruit and Nut or this Walls Chocolate Ice," but then, after a brief period, there was always a fresh pack, bottle, or ice cream and off I'd go again.

Of course I *never* saw myself as an addict. Surely that word was better matched to drugs and *serious* drinking.

Chocolate was one of my most daunting desires. I never met a chocolate candy that I didn't like (even the—in my opinion—revolting soft runny cherry liqueur candies could be swallowed whole so I could only taste the chocolate!).

I once ate the entire bottom layer of a large gift box of chocolates knowing that eventually Treena would sample the last of the first layer, lift the paper—only to find it empty. (I don't think I need to explain what happened next!)

Chocolate was only a small part of my increasing deposit of subcutaneous fat, but its contribution was *meaningful!*

I decided to arrive at a portion size that would be both reasonable and moderate for me—just me—nobody else.

I went out and bought a large bar of Kit Kat, the chocolate wafer "fingers" in a bright red pack. Its size was . . . well . . . large! The kind that are sold in movie houses—long enough to share with the whole row, or at least practice pianoforte! I broke it up into fingers, put it into a Ziploc bag, and wrote my RM (reasonable/moderate) number on the outside in permanent ink: "Two pieces a day."

By the second day, I had eaten all eight (or was it ten) pieces. Clearly I had well exceeded my own privately assessed level of moderation.

I bought a second bar and with added resolve refilled my "two pieces a day" bag. The deep freeze almost flung its door open in my face, and soon the chilled chocolate was gone once again.

I was an addict!

I made the only decision I knew how to make: I prayed for a way to stand up under the temptation and sincerely believe that I was told (internally you understand) to get it (chocolates of all kinds) out of the house.

With Treena's help we did it—*for twenty-four years.*

At the end of this period we both began to notice that I had become more than just a little judgmental about chocolate, its manufacturers, its sales messages, its packaging, and the people who ate it.

My condemnation of others was universal!

During one of our Lifestyle #9 episodes, my guest suggested that chocolate was a fine food *if* it was taken at perhaps no more than one ounce per day. He had some with him (the plain, dark variety). After twenty-four years, I took a one-ounce piece and, on camera, I ate it!

With great surprise and delight, I can tell you that I liked it, but it didn't *demand* to be consumed. Now once or twice a week I may have one ounce (or so), but I'm no longer driven and no longer critical of others who eat more than I do!

Perhaps it's because I knew I had control over it, or perhaps I knew for *certain* that I was an addict. Either way, I was free!

I know of no other way of dealing with a possible "threat" than to somehow diminish its hold by reducing both volume and frequency.

I've done this with food, drink, clothes, cars, travel. What I thought I had to have, I didn't, and when I knew that was true, I knew that I had been urged to go beyond my balancing point and had taken a firm hold of indulgence (or had it taken hold of me?).

If *indulgence* is going beyond the balance point and doing harm to both myself and, to some extent, my world, then *outdul-gence* is staying within a *measured* amount of personal consumption that brings healing to my family and again to my world.

Treena and I see this as a *lifestyle for a lifetime*—ours and others. It provides us with a daily sense of purpose. We clearly benefit every day by the great gift of good health and, in addition, as our second benefit, we have the joy of meeting truly desperate needs.

We began our own double benefit journey back in 1980 in Tacoma, Washington, and truly grasped its full meaning in 1987 when Treena's health needs *demanded* measured attention.

During these periods I have tried, repeatedly, to communicate to virtually everyone I have met the idea, which I called either *double benefit* or *outdulgence.* At a typical sound-bite level, it doesn't *connect,* largely because it calls for a degree of relinquishment of a measured amount of something we actually like (even if, in the long term, it doesn't like us!).

William Barclay, the famed Scots Bible expositor, once said that "real religion requires relinquishment." Certainly the evidence we have from Jesus' life and His notable disciples ever since would indicate this to be so.

Once the idea of converting actual predictable *harm* into tangible *healing* has sunk in, there has *always* been a clear understanding of the logic. What is usually missing, as far as we can judge, is a willingness to put the idea into practice.

I need to remind myself at this point that Treena and I feel *called* to sew the seed of the idea and are *not* to wait around to see it germinate, grow, or bear fruit; that is for others.

Perhaps you?

We are absolutely certain that if we are to teach *anything,* we must be living our message. Jesus responded to hypocrisy with uncharacteristic ferocity. I can see no reason for Him to change.

So, if you were to pass on the idea of outdulgence to others, you would need to live it.

The big question is, where to begin?

It takes some early digging to uncover possible changes, and the way you dig *really* matters. It's all a question of attitude.

You start with finding your *treats*—what you *really* enjoy—because the odds are good that you may consume them often and perhaps in pretty large portions.*

If you see these "treats" as "treasure" it will help; if you see them as "threats," you may never follow through and make a change. *We know because we've tried it that way.*

A "treat" is a "treasure" if some of its value can become a healing gift for someone else *and* become a healing device for both you and your family. Surely that *is* treasure!?

Obviously I know nothing about your treats, so in order to address this issue, I must use ours—both Treena's *and* mine— because we want to be partners-in-purpose.

It may help to explain this partnership in greater depth.

We once had a couple that we were privileged to lead to the Lord. The husband had a serious addiction to alcohol that he had fought on and off for many tragic years.

Unfortunately, his wife didn't see her occasional glass of wine at dinner as a THREAT to *her.* Indeed, for *her* it may well have been a completely acceptable TREAT. For him, however, that "innocent" glass was a tremendous temptation.

I cannot say that her habit was responsible for his harm, but I can say it wasn't a help. A partner-in-purpose needs to fully adopt the message in Romans: "It is a noble thing not to eat meat, or drink wine, or do anything that makes your brother stumble" (14:21).

When chocolate was my problem, Treena, as my partner-in-purpose, fully agreed that it wouldn't enter the house—*ever.*

I have made many food and wine decisions based upon the strength of this biblical absolute. Initially the butter, cakes, full-fat ice cream, steaks, and so forth, were reduced in portion size or replaced because of their risk to Treena (high cholesterol, hypertension, type 2 diabetes, stroke, and heart attack). By joining her in her new lifestyle, I also benefited; I lost weight, reduced a good cholesterol to very good, and feel great!

So, is this a sacrifice?

In one sense, if I was the only one that mattered, then yes! But I'm not the only one; therefore the apparent sacrifice becomes a considerable blessing—to us both.

*See Favorite Foods lists beginning on page 236.

Chapter Six

THE MEASUREMENT OF MODERATION

I am a six foot one male, Treena is five foot. I weigh between 188 and 195 pounds; Treena, 128 and 131. Obviously we don't need an identical diet, and differences such as ours occur in most families.

How then does one measure what is moderate?

Moderation can best be seen as a food/beverage intake that maintains a healthy weight, without too many ups and downs of three pounds or more. This can be measured in calories—the amount of heat needed to raise one liter (those *large* soda bottles) of water one degree centigrade.

As I write this, Treena and I are in Mt. Shasta in northern California, and the outside temperature is 37° F. My body temperature is 98.6° F; so, apart from a small electric fire and some clothes, how is it that I am sixty-one degrees hotter than it is outside? The answer, of course, is that my body is burning up calories, much like a furnace burns oil.

The calories I burn come from the food I eat.

- Carbohydrates (basically plant life) provide four calories for every one gram (the weight of a paper clip).
- Fats, of all kinds, provide nine calories for one gram.
- Protein (all "animal" life and some plants) provide four calories.
- Alcohol comes up with seven calories per gram.

Over the years that we've been measuring, we've noticed that the percentage of calories recommended to be eaten from each of these four elements has varied and may continue to do so because science is always tracking down what is *true*. However, when it comes to food intake, what may be true for you may not be for me. Because of this, the experts tend to deal in averages that *sort of fit,* but their numbers are not glove tight!

Treena and I have kept good records of our daily intake and our daily weight as well as cholesterol and blood sugar numbers, and we decided to get our calories in the following percentages:

	Daily Calories	Fat	Saturated Fat	Carbohydrates	Protein
TREENA	1,200	20%	(5%)	40%	40%
GRAHAM	2,000	20%	(5%)	50%	30%

We no longer consume alcohol because of Treena's medications and Rom. 12:21.

Of course very few people total their daily calories every day. While this can be done, it can become an obsessive-compulsive behavior, and nobody needs that!

What Treena and I did was count calories for just one typical week. We used a metric scale and a wonderful little purse-sized book called *The Doctors Pocket Calorie, Fat, and*

Carbohydrate Counter by Allan Borushck. (P.O. Box 1616, Costa Mesa, CA 92628. It's the best seven dollars you will *ever* spend.)

Once we had done our detailed homework for just one week, we discovered we could weigh portions of foods with our eyes! We had won the battle by making a presumptive strike where it most matters. *Calories are important!*

When we had our portion sizes moderated, we took an honest look at what we actually ate at one typical "sitting" of the foods we *really* enjoyed. We called this our "favorite foods assessment list," and we've included this as an appendix in this book starting on page 236.

I'm not going to plead with you because I really don't think it would help, but please forgive me if I become somewhat passionate about the list! Our entire theory of outdulgence (to convert a harmful habit into a healing resource) depends upon *each of us* asking ourselves the hard questions needed in order to complete the list. It's really the only way we've found to target our balance point—that amount we consume that we need for good health and beyond which we overconsume on our way to predictable chronic disease.

I admit that it takes a lot of patience. It took us many hours to assemble and test it, but we've been quite pleased with the results because

- We have found an *individual* way of measuring what is moderate.
- By our daily journal entries, we can check that it's working (see pp. 246–47).
- We have projected what our annual savings would be, and because of those totals, we adjusted our budget for food and our giving by the exact amounts we projected. This has helped us to stay faithful to our carefully made decisions.
- We really have reduced our overall consumption, and we can see the *measurable* benefits to our daily health and sense of well-being.

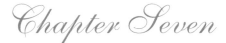

PREVENTION OR PROTECTION

Often I act to *prevent* something from happening. The best example must surely be totally giving up smoking in order to prevent lung cancer, heart disease, emphysema, or even wrinkled facial skin and bad breath!

We *prevent* a predictable disease or disfigurement.

The word *protect* is somewhat different and carries with it the sense of defending against a predictable attack of some kind. I can, for example, *protect* my skin by using sunscreen, but that is also a means of prevention of both skin cancers and wrinkles (not a real "guy" problem!).

Protection, in the way I want to use it here, is an absolutely vital prelude to the selection of a lifestyle that I can live for a lifetime. For such a long-lasting selection to be made, I must be focused on the *defense* of something of utmost value to me—and that isn't just my health, as important as that may be.

I need to protect my *self-worth*! I need to build it and protect it because it is vulnerable to all kinds of attack.

At its most simplistic level, when I stand on the scales and my weight has gone up a pound or so, my self-worth suffers (especially if I *know* what did it!).

When I had a disturbed night's sleep following a marathon of TV viewing, my self-worth suffered.

When I used to take just one small drink, and I knew it didn't work for me, my self-worth suffered!

Somehow I knew, deep down inside, that what I chose to do was harming me, and yet I chose to do it in spite of that still small voice of warning inside.

When I smother the inner voice of reason, I believe I directly subtract from my "store" of self-worth. I make a deficit decision that actually weakens my overall resolve to change my ways. Eventually even my willingness to consider a positive change suffers. When there is little self-worth, why bother to protect it!

This is why I see our self-worth as vulnerable. If it can be progressively weakened, then whatever witness we have becomes invalid as we become an invalid.

My poet-wife Treena once wrote a beautiful poem to describe her early search for self-worth and its value.

Self-Worth

I wandered lonely through the fields
whilst searching for a worth in self.
I saw fresh leaves upon old trees;
wild flowers dressing fields anew
brought butterflies of every hue,
each uniquely individual.

The smallest wing, the tiniest petal
each so delicately settled.
Perfection—Worth a lingering stare.
Nature's self-worth was everywhere.

I stirred upon the rugged fence
on which I sat and there did muse,
"I too am fashioned by the Hand
that has created nature's way!"
Suddenly—a restless breeze breathed
a solace prayer into my heart,

"The secret of mankind's self-worth
is through the searching soul's rebirth.
Believe and trust in Me, my child,
My inward care will soon disclose—
all creation is divine;
though nature's breathless beauty blinds,
nothing compares with 'humankind!'"

With heart and soul restored in Him,
escorted by the Comforter—
I returned, fixed in Love and hope
to wander lonely never more—
for now, I knew His original intent,
was to be His humble instrument
that lays close by His feet to use
for those that need Him introduced.

We really do have value, and our self-worth needs protection.

I used the Collins New World Dictionary of the American Language as a first-level word search and went looking for *self-worth* only to find it missing. There are 197 words with the hyphenated "self" as a compound, from *self-abasement* to *self-will,* but no *self-worth!* The dictionary does describe *worth* as "that quality of a person (or thing) that lends importance, value, merit, etc., and that is *measurable* by the esteem in which the person or thing is held" (italics mine).

All of this led me to conclude that *self-worth* needs to be *measured* by some means—yet not by others, but by me.

I was struck by the phrase in the definition "that quality of a person" and reflected upon the qualities described in Paul's letter to the Galatians when he described the fruit of the Spirit.

Love
Joy
Peace
Patience
Goodness
Kindness
Faithfulness
Gentleness
Self-Control

If I were to *measure* these on a scale of one through ten, with Jesus Christ as the example of a perfect ten, then where would I be—honestly and, yes, prayerfully—in such a measurement?

And no matter where the truth fell or how small the number, was I in fact grateful for that fruitfulness being present in my life, with its potential for growth *if I am willing*?

I settled on these *nine* qualities as worth protecting from lifestyle choices that would appear to attack them. Why, for example, do I get impatient or even unkind, and why do I lack self-control when under pressure? Most likely I'm responding to outside circumstances, choices that I've made that subtract from my store of nine self-worth qualities.

These are my deficit decisions, or my habits that harm.

I have now had thirty years to ponder what all of this might mean as Treena and I have set out to find a lifestyle for a lifetime—a set of simple measurements that can build up our self-worth (also well-being) for the rest of our lives.

It all begins with the issue of greatest value—our *witness* as influenced by the nine fruits of the spirit. This compound must be defended by all practical means and by all the spiritual disciplines we are gifted to exercise.

We have finally settled upon four major "strong towers" of lifestyle defense.

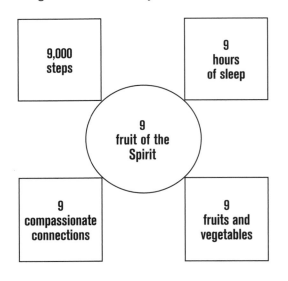

The measurement of *nine* in each case is not just a matter of mathematic simplicity. It is meant to focus attention upon the *nine/self-worth*. It also suggests that the perfection of ten may well be beyond anyone's reach! But there is also strong scientific support for the physical activity of nine thousand steps, nine hours of sleep, and nine servings of fruit and vegetables.

Treena and I have also proved (to ourselves) that our nine compassionate connections are vitally important to keep us on track (consistent) while our old habits begin to fade.

Whenever we share this simple formula: $9 + 9 + 9 + 9 = 9$, we urge people to be really honest about where they are each day and to consider how they may advance to the next numbers without any form of legalism (which we see as deadly to the whole idea because it is self-righteousness!).

If you eat three servings of fruit and vegetables per day (as do most Americans) then try for four or perhaps five and keep the ultimate in mind. *Any progress you make will add to your sense of self-worth* and will also protect against choices that could subtract from the self-same storehouse of real value.

For nine self-tests of self-worth, please turn to page 248.

Chapter Eight

BETWEEN A ROCK AND A HARD PLACE

For several years, from 1971 to 2004, Treena and I were sailors. We covered roughly thirty thousand miles in several sailboats and enjoyed the peace, the freedom, and to a lesser extent, the moments of tension. One of those tense moments serves well to illustrate my first point on where to choose to change . . .

We were a good five miles from a safe harbor when a sudden gale hit us. What seemed to be a relatively easy approach between a rocky shoal and the narrow harbor entry was being swept by an ugly swell.

Tension set in; decisions had to be made. Would we go in closer and try to enter, or go about and slog it out for another twenty miles to hopefully find a more protected anchorage?

We kept on our course as I checked and double-checked the chart. On a fine day, it would have been tight yet quite easy, but today. . . .

We dropped our sails, turned on the engine, and began to pitch violently as we closed. We could see the rocks and the harbor wall. We'd have to go between a rock and a very hard place.

We were committed and had to turn broadside to the breaking swell and use every ounce of power our engine would give us. We rolled savagely, our mast whipping by overhead like a metronome in a heavy-metal rock concert.

The harbor wall beat back the waves, and they met in spouts where the entrance lay. We both wore life jackets and lifelines shackled to the cockpit sole, but it felt beyond control and the wind shrieked as we charged through the spray.

Suddenly it was over. We were in flat, sheltered water as I swiftly reversed the engine to save colliding with the tiny harbormasters dock.

We were safe, we did it! Yeah!

So, what on earth does this have to do with choosing how to eat?

When we are quite young—let's say all the way from eighteen to fifty—we are several miles out from the "coast" and any possible "physical" difficulty. The idea of planning in advance for a problem doesn't seem to make much sense.

But as the coastline (increasing age) comes closer, and especially as conditions may change, we may feel the tension build.

The truth is, unless we make some wise choices when we are "out there," we may have to face making a run between a rock and a hard place—between heart disease and the increasingly obvious diabetes.

Treena and I were thirty-four when we began to make the *Galloping Gourmet* series 21 for international television. *We were way out at sea!*

Those who were wiser and closer to the "coastline" warned us of the rocks ahead, but we simply couldn't see that far, so we "galloped" on under full sail.

We eventually came to understand. The sudden storm of heart disease and stroke hit us first. All we wanted was to reach a safe harbor and be well again–*as quickly as possible.*

We have made it to that small anchorage through a passageway of hypertension, diabetes, and a triple bypass–a crosscurrent of tension and even fear.

We are now the so-called wiser ones, who have successfully weathered the storm and are urgently trying to tell those we meet who are still miles from the coastline that they also may face the need to navigate the treacherous passage now being undertaken by millions who never thought this day would come, who especially hadn't thought that there might have been a storm during their final approach.

We are now living in an extraordinary time: the baby boom generation is reaching fifty. The coastline is in sight; there are decisions to be made. Fourteen thousand boomers are reaching fifty *today* and will continue to do so day after day until 2024. Five million every year!

They each have a choice to make: will they risk the narrow entry between heart disease and diabetes and pray there is no storm, or will they pursue their goals in the hopes of finding a sheltered anchorage without the slightest difficulty.

It really is about the closing coastline. As Christians, we know that the only truly safe haven we have is when we go "home." But what about the last days of our journey? Does it have to be between a rock and a hard place during a sudden storm?

One of our guest scientists in the DVD series *Lifestyles #9* suggests that, in his opinion, roughly nine percent of all chronic diseases, such as heart disease and adult onset diabetes, could be proven to be genetic and therefore inescapable. This number suggested that behavior could account for as much as 70 percent (allowing for a 20% area open to doubt, which is Treena's background).

Let's say that most of your family has been somewhat heavy and therefore more likely to be at risk for heart disease, stroke, hypertension, and type 2 diabetes. Does that mean that those diseases are inevitable?

It depends on the food your family consumed and the quantity. In *some* cases, the potential chronic diseases such as type 2 diabetes do *appear* to be genetic, but in others it can be from observed behavior–a repeat performance of what Mom and Dad ate . . . and ate often.

Breaking such a strong cultural set of preferences is often very difficult because a family food preference is interwoven with all kinds of other mostly pleasant memories. Families often find themselves in the *same boat,* facing a predictable storm as their coastline of age approaches.

The facts prove, for the most part, that we do not have to remain in that boat. We can do our part to avoid, or at least better manage, our exposure to chronic disease, and that change can be remarkably effective!

We know because Treena got out of her family boat and jumped into mine, which, with its "gourmet" behavior, wasn't much better! But eventually we made the right choices and found a lifestyle we could live for a lifetime—and it's working!

Right choices are not, however, an open ticket to longevity. A long life isn't always a blessing. What does matter in the long run is one's ability to keep moving with a real God-given purpose, a reason to be alive and as well as possible.

A British minister of health originally coined the phrase, "It's not more years in your life, its more life in your years." This is especially so for us as Christians. We may well have risen with wings as eagles, or have run without being weary, but eventually we must be content to walk without becoming faint (see Isa. 40:31).

It is during this less-frenetic "walk" that we may best encounter the measured pace of Jesus and, as we move to find ourselves, be better able to both understand and communicate the kingdom of God.

But what if we can no longer walk, and what if pain or discomfort so fully occupies our days that we have little time to consider our ongoing usefulness even as prayer warriors for those in greater distress than ourselves?

The chances are that you are still *out at sea*—there is still time to make some well-considered choices before the time of "faltering" arrives.

If so, then what might your choices be?

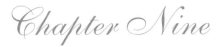

HOW WE JUMPED SHIP

Treena and I had our epiphany when she had her heart attack back in November 1987, during a University of the Nations course on leadership in Kona, Hawaii. Four months before that she had a stroke and also had seriously elevated cholesterol.

The emergency room physician in Hawaii bluntly advised, "Make your peace with her. By looking at her EKG, I don't think she can pull through this."

We flew from Kona to Honolulu in an air ambulance, and it was there that we made our decision to change. For her part, Treena, in a maze of wires and IVs, looked at my worried face and thought, "Why didn't I do what he said?" And I, in the deepest known upheaval of my entire life was saying, "Why did I make it all so difficult? If there's a second chance, I'll do it right. Lord, please let there be a second chance!"

Our thoughts and prayers were answered. We were given three months to see if a change of lifestyle could make enough difference to avoid surgical intervention.

Together we jumped ship.

That was in December 1987.

Suddenly, a violent storm arose on the sea, so that the boat was being swamped by the waves. But He was sleeping. So the disciples came and woke Him up, saying, "Lord save us! We're going to die!"

But He said to them, "Why are you fearful, you of little faith?" Then He got up and rebuked the winds and the sea. And there was a great calm. (Matt. 8:24–26 HCSB)

We had been fearful, we had certainly called out to the Lord to help us, and I can admit to being quite low in faith.

But there came a great calm.

I found a small excerpt from the written works of John of the Cross, a monk who served in Spain in and around 1420. It reads: "If you love someone you do them good and the good you do them you do with the best in your nature." Without doubt, the *best in my nature* was now Jesus: "I have been crucified with Christ, and I no longer live, but Christ lives in me" (Gal. 2:19–20).

In the midst of our sudden storm, Jesus guided us between the rock and the hard place, and our faith (no matter how little) was our life jacket and safety line.

We learned to live creatively and gradually to set aside the past habits that had, in part, caused us harm.

As I look back on those remarkable days of change, there is no doubt as to the sequence. The first "baby" step was one of *attitude* and had nothing to do with food! Before, I had been fully convinced that we could find the best of health by *avoiding* certain obviously risky foods. I set up a style of eating for our family based upon "thou shalt not . . ."

One of my multiple problems, along with self-righteousness and the desire to control, was my *absolutism.* If something *appeared* to be risky, it was history. I invented an exclusionary diet, full of my rules. I would tolerate no argument. I knew better because I'd read all the little diet books and had developed a real food phobia.

Eventually, if you build a big enough barricade, you'll get a rebellion, and that's exactly what had happened to me (you can read about this rebellion in our book *Recipe for Life*).

Finally I agreed to a compromise in the face of total rebellion: I'd cook two meals— one for the rebels, the other for good old clean-living me!

It was eight years after this infantile behavior that Treena entered her storms of stroke and heart attack. She was fifty-three, too young to die! But her troubles had begun way back in 1974 when I discovered legalism and then compounded my error with compromise.

It was this attitude that had to change and change *first.* Without a sincere change of heart, all the best external choices in the world may only lead to legalism, which, in the long run, is deadly.

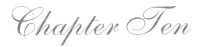

OUR DAY-BY-DAY ATTITUDE

In the old days, Treena and I were often asked, "Who does the cooking in your house?" That question has now been superceded by "What do you eat on a typical day?"

The reason for the switch is, we believe, because of the relative success we've had with our now "settled" lifestyle. It's as though people want us to develop a diet based on our day-by-day experiences!

I've always tried to resist this temptation, mostly because almost everyone nowadays seems to have a diet that "works for them"—that is, for a while.

I'm inclined to think that the word *diet* should be replaced by the word *attitude.* With a positive attitude based on a known need—such as weight loss, cholesterol, or blood pressure reductions—all that's needed is to find a practical example of what has been proven to work for someone we trust.

Since you are reading *this* book, it is our hope (no, it's our prayer!) that something we do may seem to you to be attractive enough to be given a try.

In a normal "brief encounter" (are you old enough to remember that movie?) we don't usually have the time to properly describe a typical day, whatever *that* is! However, given your present *attitude* of inquiry and the space we have in this book, I'm able to give you a complete answer.

Before we begin let me remind you that this is not a restrictive diet, but rather a way of life—a lifestyle to be modified to suit *your* circumstances and then, hopefully, to be maintained as a lifetime example for others to observe.

Our day-by-day "choices" are based on one idea, or attitude: We convert *any* habit that harms us into a resource that heals others.

The famed American jurist Oliver Wendell Holmes once said, "I wouldn't give you a fig for simplicity this side of complexity but I would give my life for simplicity on the other side of complexity."

We've named his goal OSOC for *other side of complexity,* and that has been our attitude—to live more simply, not for our sake alone but for what that can mean as an encouragement to others.

We began with the usual *us first* focus because it was so often promoted in media that we simply couldn't escape it! Yet when we took to heart the idea of *loving our neighbors as ourselves,* we developed a whole new attitude toward lifestyle choices. It would, from then on, always be us *and* them—a lifestyle for a lifetime!

Our second building block of attitude was the word *treat,* which we've discussed before. The word *treat* ends in *eat,* and we sincerely believe that it should be a treat to eat and not a *threat,* which also ends in *eat!*

The difference in the two words is the letter H, which stands for *high* in volume (portion size) and high in repetition (frequency of selection). By *always* considering both portion size and frequency, we continually adjust our consumption directly to our need.

A change of habit usually means smaller portions chosen less frequently, and that *usually* means we spend less on our day-by-day food budget. What we save (which used to harm us) can now heal someone else—*if we keep our eyes open for those in need.* If we don't have an eye for our neighbors, then the savings often go to purchase the next best thing, or to pay off a debt, or be saved for a good use (child's education, etc.).

There is nothing *wrong* with personal expenditures that benefit ones own family. What we are proposing, however, is to transfer what you are now spending in time and money on something that specifically *harms* you and/or your family and to convert exactly that time or money to a cause that somehow provides healing for our often desperate global neighbors. You will benefit (a harmful habit changed) and so will someone else! It's not all about you or me or us—it's also about *them!*

Frankly, it's often enormously hard to step out of the normal commercial flow of choices and consume less, but we've found that it's possible in the long term (a lifestyle for a lifetime) when you feel connected to someone else by a deliberate compassionate choice.

Our meat *choices* connect us to Sadik in Ethiopia. Treena's latte's, to Nicaragua; her

decorative nails, to Africa. Our cheese, to Bellevue, Washington, teens. Our cookies, to Brazil. The list goes on and on.

Almost always we don't cut things out; we reduce them from threat to treat.

To help you address this amazing source of potential generosity, I've included a list of treats, starting on page 236, that can easily become threats. If I told you what was a "good" portion size, I would introduce a new set of legalisms and utterly destroy the whole idea of outdulgence. In order for outdulgence to work and to multiply, the entire concept must be grounded in *love.* Love of God, love of neighbor, love of self with all our heart, soul, mind, and strength.

This is what it means to be human in the best possible sense, and it's based upon an inner attitude and not a restrictive *diet* of anything!

~ ~ ~

So now, given that foundation, let's take a look at our typical day.

Firstly, a glance at the big picture:

6:00–7:30	Quiet time (toast and tea)
7:30–8:30	Prayer walk and stretch
9:00–9:30+	Breakfast
11:00–11:15	Fruit or fruit snack
1:00–1:45	Lunch (often the main meal of the day)
4:00	Afternoon tea (tea, crisp bread)
6:00–7:00	Dinner (mostly "nibbles"– see p. 230)
8:30	Bedtime snack (small milk, cookie)
9:00	Bed

Within this context we try to

- eat 9 servings of fruit and vegetables
- walk 9,000 steps
- sleep 9 hours
- provide for 9 people-groups from our savings of time and money

Our success is not based *entirely* on weight loss and health or on people helped but upon the gradual maturing of these nine words: love, joy, peace, patience, goodness, kindness, faithfulness, gentleness, self-control.

That is our reward!

Now it's time to cut to the chase and begin to lay out pages of special helps and recipes for you. Keep in mind that *each recipe is a guide.* Should you dislike an ingredient (such as anchovies), you may want to replace it with capers or some other intense seasoning that *you* enjoy!

To help you fully understand your personal preferences, please read the instructions and complete the Food Preference Sheets, starting on page 249. It will take only one hour to provide you with a very real tool to upgrade almost every recipe ever written and make it *yours!*

Now, let us begin!

SPECIAL HELPS

BUYING

1. Fruits and Vegetables. I always think about plant life in order of its degree of excellence, both in flavor and nutrition. Best are those we grow ourselves organically from heirloom seeds known for the best flavor, like the Brandywine tomato and the new hybrid Viva Italia (blight resistant and great taste for cooking).

My next level is the local organic farmer with a roadside stand or a booth at the Farmer's Market—even in the midst of Manhattan at Union Square. If you look for them, you'll find them; they keep increasing because they are the lifeblood of the small farmer, and they are well worth supporting.

Strangely, I often find that frozen vegetables come next because the best suppliers harvest and process within a twenty-four- to forty-eight-hour period. The fresh supplies in the best supermarkets may be better but not always. And then there is the "normal" market where the produce may have been trucked more than 1,800 miles and be days old.

Finally, there's canned or bottled, which is storage convenient and sometimes excellent, such as canned tomato pastes and sauces and light-syrup or water-packed fruit.

This logically brings us to canned soups, which I use quite often but never simply as they are made. I enhance these soups with taste, aroma, color, and texture (T.A.C.T.). Take a look at Tactful Soup, p. 63, and you'll get the idea.

I usually buy Progresso soups and mostly their mixed vegetable combinations since we prefer to add our own protein. Watch for summer specials, especially down South. It's a great time to stock up, and they keep well (see Tactful Soup, p. 63.)

2. Filtered Water. We have now spent many a year both sailing and recently "camping" in our motor home. Early on, we encountered "odd" water supplies, mostly overchlorinated. When the water content of a dish is large (for example, tea and some soups—see p. 66, Tomato Soup with a Twist) then the chlorine *has* to go. But how? We found the BRITA filter system and its one quart jug and have used this with great success for more than two years. We refill the jug at least three times a day and change the filter once every three months. Compared to bottled water, it's a great buy.

1221 Broadway
Oakland, CA 94612
1-800-24-BRITA

3. Nonaromatic Olive Oil. I use this phrase throughout the book whenever I need a *little* good oil to sauté (fry). Because I use so little and because the heat (acting on such a small quantity) drives off the fragrance of extra-virgin olive oils, I have chosen an oil by Bertolli that they call "Extra-Light." This means *light* in flavor because all oil is 9 calories for each 1 gram and it cannot be *lightened* in its nutritional "fats" content.

Because it is *nonaromatic* (the term I prefer to avoid confusion), it is also less expensive but still an excellent choice for *all* culinary tasks, except perhaps for salads and some seafood, where a very good extra-virgin olive oil (kept in a cool dark place but the fridge at 40°F is too cold) will do splendidly.

4. Low-Fat Sausages. Whenever we use sausage, we try to find those that combine low-fat with increased flavor. There are few nationally available brands, and those that use turkey as the meat tend to be too bland. We go for those with the description "Italian"; the ones that use a chicken base seem best (see Leaf Greens and Sausage over Pasta, p. 71).

5. Parmesan Cheese. For years I purchased the famed Italian original Parmegianno Reggiano, always in a piece I kept wrapped in a clean piece of cheesecloth soaked in a little white wine vinegar. I now buy Wisconsin Parmesan, which I store in the same way and freshly grate when needed. The cost is almost 50 percent less! As for the cheap, already grated parmesan, it simply doesn't deliver enough good flavor when used one tablespoon at a time, so more is added and the economic benefit is lost!

6. Pastas. It is true that whole wheat pastas provide a slight benefit with the use of whole grain and fiber, and these would seem to slow down the conversion of starch to sugar. However, since my portion sizes call for no more than 2 ounces "raw" weight (uncooked), the benefit is so slight that I've had to compare it to the quality achieved with the classic Durum semolina. To my taste the classic wins! It is also, in most cases, less expensive.

7. The Poële Method. This method uses hard root vegetables and is therefore the perfect method for those blustery, cold winter days when the hard squash, turnips, parsnips, and rutabaga are all at their best and least expensive. This is a fine way to reach toward the nine servings of fruit and vegetables we *need* every day (see Poële, pp. 78, 80).

8. Herbs of Provence. You will find that this particular blend of dried herbs is widely stocked in most supermarkets. While the blending is a little different depending upon the packager, it is usually a blend of bay leaf, thyme, rosemary, basil, and lavender—all highly aromatic. As with any herb, I use *just* enough and no more—more is *never* better with herbs. I use it often to reduce the need to buy jar after jar of "single" herbs that often get used once and then spoil (lose their flavor). They have become, for me, a special "family" flavor that sets apart dishes created during the past three years (see Poële, p. 78).

I have also re-introduced my ETHMIX™ range of regional seasonings in culinary leaf form (rather than the previous powdered line). These can be ordered at www.graham kerr.com or www.daybydaygourmet.com.

9. Barley. This comes in two styles: pearl and pot. The *pearl* cooks quicker, but the *pot* has more texture and stands up better when cooked in soups and stews (see Barley, p. 91).

10. Quinoa. This seed grain is a great side dish and *just* edges out couscous as the lightest grain at 83 calories for 1/2 cup (see p. 92).

11. Long-Grain Brown Rice. Sure it takes longer to cook (twice the time, actually), but you get added texture and flavor, plus it takes longer to absorb into the bloodstream, making it a wise choice for diabetics and weight loss (see p. 93). I have *very* recently found a Minute Brown Rice (precooked) that retains its texture and nutrition.

12. Angel Hair Pasta (Whole Wheat). As a rule, I prefer the hard Durum semolina wheat pasta because of its "quality" texture. An exception can be made with the fine Angel Hair, where the size allows the whole wheat to be less intrusive (see p. 95).

13. Wild Mushrooms. These are usually "wildly" expensive unless you try this simple and *eventually* convenient idea. Buy dried mushrooms, usually in 1/2-oz. packages. I get chanterelles, morel, oyster, and shitake—Frieda's brand is very good.

I then whiz them into a fine powder in a high-speed coffee grinder (clean it first!).

I keep the powder in a plastic bag in the fridge and use only one level teaspoon for each 1/2 pound of regular mushrooms. I get just enough "wild" flavor to satisfy (see p. 96) at a fraction of the cost.

14. Tomato Spaghetti Sauce. A *well-made* marinara styled spaghetti sauce is an excellent example of a processed food that really works. The flavor is good and little to no harm is done in processing. Just be care-

ful to note the sodium content (see Spaghetti Squash, p. 99).

15. The Idaho or Russet Potato. Easily the best for baking and certainly the best for my "Diamond in the Jacket" (p. 103). Be careful to buy the smaller russets (about 3 inches long); some of the larger ones can pack in extra calories that we don't need.

16. Fingerling Potatoes. Here is another example of quality versus sheer size. The fingerling is a "skin-and-all" edible root quite like a waxy, creamy new potato except that it is small sausage shaped (see p. 88). We serve no more than two to three ounces per head, which adds up to 50 percent less than the average potato side-dish portion.

17. Refreshing Seafood. There is a Scottish Island technique that "refreshes" or "revives" seafood that has been out of the sea for a *few* hours (by no means is this idea to be used on old, poorly handled fish for which there should be no sale!). Dissolve a little sea salt in ice cold water until it tastes like sea water. Cover the fish in this chilled "sea water" for fifteen minutes. Remove. Dry on paper towels and then cook immediately. Good fish will be even better than ever (see Tilapia, p. 107).

18. Tilapia. This is now a well-established fresh, farm-raised fish like trout, salmon, and catfish. A native of Israel, it has been fished commercially for more than two thousand years.

It has been my fish of preference for several reasons. It is always fresh on a good seafood counter and seldom "previously frozen." It is a firm-textured white fish that is bone free (obviously when filleted). It does not have a pronounced "fishy" aroma. Finally, it has the clean crisp taste you associate with good fish. I've used it to show how fish are breaded and pan fried (p. 107), poached (p. 113), and baked (p. 111).

19. Wine. You will notice that I use a selection of de-alcoholized wines in my recipes. I do this because to my taste they are better. Often, when using wines with alcohol, you will be asked to heat the wine to "evaporate" the alcohol. This effectively reduces the alcohol "texture" or bite (because alcohol has neither aroma nor flavor), the "burn" to the mouth that can unbalance a good sauce.

I use a wine made as a good wine should be. Then the alcohol is removed by reverse osmosis, during which the smallest molecules (water and alcohol) are removed. Water is replaced, and the now "de-alcoholized" wine is bottled.

Sutter Homes Fre is widely available in supermarkets and tends to "hide out" on the bottom shelf of the lower-cost Californian wines. *Ask and you may find!*

I've come to value these wines without alcohol, especially because of the Scripture that requires me to do *nothing* by which "your brother stumbles or is offended or is made weak" (Rom. 14:22 KJV).

I use my own techniques of "splashing" a dish at the last moment in order to obtain a fresh wine finish that previously boiled wine cannot have because it has lost some of its *aromas* in the boiling process. The Merlot and Premium White by Fre are my usual purchases (see Baked White Fish, p. 114).

20. Salmon. I am well aware of the controversy surrounding "farmed" versus "wild" salmon. For day-to-day eating I am content with farmed. My extensive research has led me to conclude that those I love are in no risk from the consumption (and the price is right). I also know that it has not been previously frozen. For special occasions I seek out—*in season*—the best of the Pacific wild king cohos (Copper River, etc.). Costing up to four times the farmed salmon, the extraordinary richness in omega 3 fatty acids and other wild food flavors make them almost a completely different fish (see Poached Salmon, p. 122).

21. Fish Sauce. Nam pla (Thailand), patis (Philippines), shottsura (Japan), and nuoc nam (Vietnam)—all are very salty, very fishy, thin dark liquids often used in place of salt as a general flavor base for Southeast Asian dishes. Somewhat of an acquired aroma but well worth the try.

22. Canadian Bacon (Pea meal in Canada!). In numerous classical cuisines, bacon, fat back and even cured pork fat is used for its marvelous rich, salty, smooth-textured contribution. Unfortunately, it can be overdone, delivering levels of saturated fat, sodium, and nitrates that we find hard to handle.

I use very small amounts of the very lean Canadian or "back" bacon cut quite fine in order to well distribute its taste. 1/2 oz. per head is usually just enough (see Braised Chicken with Pasta, p. 165).

23. Chicken. At the time of this writing, I'm having an argument with myself over the use of growth hormones, antibiotics, and the mass-crowding of battery-raised chickens. There is nothing that I like about this high intensive "farming" system—*other than* *the price!* But is there a *real* risk? If there is, wouldn't free-range/organic be a worthwhile "upgrade" (or perhaps consuming more vegetables and not buying flesh protein at all!)?

24. Chicken Thighs versus Breasts. If a dish is to be presented in one piece, then the breast wins hands down because it *looks better.* If the dish calls for moist heat braising or stewing or is a casserole, then the more collagen content (connective tissues) is far better than the often dry, chewiness of the breast. The stir-fry still favors the breast, but be very careful not to overcook (see Chicken Stir-Fry, Thai Style, p. 163).

25. Chicken Breast–Skinless (see also Culinary Techniques). In its effort to meet the lower fat demands of the consumer, the poultry industry decided to remove the breast skin. "Skinless Chicken Breasts" apparently sell better–but they don't cook better! The skin helps to retain moisture, so I buy my chickens (free range!) whole and do my own cutting. I save money, and I get the skin, which I discard when the breast is cooked (see Curried Chicken, p. 173).

26. Coconut. One of my favorite *treats* is the coconut cream used in southern Indian and Thai dishes, as well as elsewhere throughout the tropics. Unfortunately, it does come complete with substantial saturated fat content. I need to keep saturated fat levels to 7 percent or less of total calories to avoid the effect on LDL cholesterol.

While coconut could be of little real impact unless used frequently, my sense is always to try to find alternatives. Every small "allowance" will eventually add up and become a potential consequence–especially for someone with increased risk, like Treena. Because of this I've experimented with adding coconut flavor oil to my yogurt cheese and thickened stock (see p. 37). I've also used the Coconut Milk Lite that now comes canned. I can't go all the way with the full-on Coconut Cream and still keep a recipe out of what I see (for our personal health needs) as harm's way (see Chicken Stir-fry, Thai Style, p. 163).

Also, I discovered Lorann Gourmet Coconut Oil flavor as a reasonable replacement for my favorite Wagner's Coconut Essence, which, regrettably, went out of business. It can be used like vanilla in small doses for big flavors.

For the creaminess I use one of my yogurt cheese sauces (see p. 38). It works quite well in comfort dishes where it delivers both the aroma and texture of the original–but it's fat-free (see Hawaiian Curried Chicken, p. 140).

27. Tomato Paste and Depth of Flavor. "Fat adds flavor" is a true statement, but that doesn't mean you must add it (or that you can't remove some of it). Other things also add flavor, amongst which is one of my favorites: tomato paste.

The flavor comes when the paste is cooked over a high heat and spread about the pan base so that the natural sugars caramelize (brown). This takes 5 minutes or so of constant stirring, but the results are spectacular! I use this when I need both flavor depth and that deep rich mahogany color that fine beef stews have (see Steak and Oyster Pie, p. 180, and the Blade Steak and Beer Stew, p. 184, as only two of many examples).

28. Datil Pepper. This unique pepper, native to Portugal, was brought over by the folks who founded the city of St. Augustine. It is still grown in Florida but is not as widely distributed as the Jalapeño or Anaheim.

29. Low-Cost Cooked Meat. The lowest cost meat I've found is the picnic shoulder, which in my case worked out to only $2.50 (U.S.) per pound when all fat and bone was removed. The problem is that you are left with untidy little slices; therefore, the better use is as shredded pork often found in Mexican dishes. I like the flavor, and because we use only 2 to 3 ounces per head in such dishes, it seems like a good investment. (Please see all the details at Roast Pork Picnic Shoulder, p. 195, and watch out for the crackling!)

30. Southeast Asian Chile Paste. This almost "lethal" vividly hot spice paste comes in a glass jar (presumably because it could eat through an aluminum can!). It is the means by which most Asian restaurants graduate "spice heat" from one star to five, and only a small amount is needed. When opened, it must be refrigerated. Buy in small quantities unless you have an "asbestos mouth" (see Spicy Pork and Potato Casserole, p. 202).

31. Lemon Grass. This herb grows well in California and has a long tight almost "woody" stem with a tender tip. The wider the stem's diameter, the tougher the slice. I like to grate it, or at least very finely slice the more tender tops. It is acidic (like lemon) but more herbal than fruity (see Chicken Stir-Fry, Thai Style, p. 163).

32. Pumpkin Cheese Flatbread. This is so good that I'm giving you the address—what we used to call an "unsolicited testimonial." One cracker is 100 calories, 11 grams carbohydrates with 4 grams fiber. Net carbs per slice is 8—and they taste wonderful! Completely organic. The brand is Dr. Kracker (10490 Milles Rd., Dallas, TX 57238). Also, see Composed "Fruited" Salad on page 70.

33. Phyllo (also filo or fillo) is an extremely thin dough that is layered to produce a flaky pastry. As a substitute for a pie crust, the new whole wheat phyllo can be used to greatly reduce both fat and carbs. I suggest the organic whole wheat phyllo from

The Fillo Factory
www.fillofactory.com
Dumont, NJ 07628

NUTRITION

I simply can't let this section's notes on nutrition begin without discussing portion size. The western developed world has now officially recognized that obesity, and to a slightly less extent overweight, is a global threat.

To be markedly overweight is a disease that can lead to heart disease, type 2 diabetes, and some cancers. Add in hypertension, chronic digestive diseases, and painful wear and tear on joints, and it's no big surprise that the experts are concerned. Perhaps the greatest concern lies in the *fact* that the solution is so simple, yet so apparently hard to apply. In its stripped down format it says:

EAT LESS AND MOVE MORE
or
FEWER CALORIES IN
AND MORE CALORIES OUT

To apply this solution means that you *must* find a way to count calories, both in and out. Frankly, that takes diligence—I know because I've spent thousands of hours over the past thirty-three years doing exactly that.

As calories are reduced, so are portion sizes. In this book they've reached what we call an RM level. RM stands for *reasonable moderate,* and it is different according to individual needs.

A fairly major difference exists between my overall plate appearance and that provided by many of today's restaurants. The protein element is less, as is the starch-based carbohydrates. The vegetables on the other hand have been substantially increased.

Eating this way will be *different,* and that's going to be your first hurdle! You must remember that most of us eat too much, so in order to reduce that quantity, the portions *must* get smaller.

1. Fall and Winter. When the keen northern winds pick up in the fall, we enjoy the more robust soups—ones that use the winter crops of hard storable "root" vegetables and winter squash (pumpkin, butternut, acorn, etc.). When deeply colored vegetables are used (carrot, sweet potato) the Vitamin A levels can be extraordinary, and the natural fiber deducted from total carbohydrate is less responsive, so there is slower blood sugar increase (see FABIS: The Cream of Soups, p. 64).

2. F.A.B.I.S. This acronym stands for Fresh And Best In Season. There is no better choice for flavor and nutrition and celebrating the seasons as the new crops arrive. A simple way to test this is to cook two ears of corn together (wrap in paper towel and microwave for 4 minutes on full power). Let the first ear be the new season's off the local farm, and the second, one that you purchased from a "normal" store. Chew on each and you'll get the message. And, of course, all this will add wonderfully to your nine servings of fruit and vegetables a day.

3. Serving Sizes of Fruit and Vegetables. It's easy to say nine *servings,* but few people we meet have any idea what that means (another example of sound bytes with no depth of understanding). So here's the answer:

Leafy greens (pressed in tight)	1 cup =	1 serving
Chopped hard vegetable (i.e., carrot)	1/2 cup =	1 serving
100% fruit juice	3/4 cup =	1 serving
Medium-sized whole fruit	1 =	1 serving
Dried fruit	1/4 cup =	1 serving

I hope, when you see this, that the idea of "nine a day" doesn't look so daunting.

4. Fiber. By now most of us have heard that fiber is a good idea. It eases the digestive and evacuation process, and it slows down carbohydrate/sugar absorption for diabetics as well as reducing adverse LDL cholesterol. So, when fiber crops up in a splendid salad with 12 grams, it's well worth a try (see Spinach Salad, p. 69).

5. Tortillas. These very useful and enjoyable "breads" come in a variety of sizes and content. In a very general way, they come either as "flour" or "corn" and, more recently, whole grains are being used as well as that magic "upgrade": *organic!* You should know that the 6-inch corn usually weighs 1.2 ounces and has 45 calories, 5 grams of fat, and 9 grams of carbohydrates compared to the wheat flour version that weighs 1.75 ounces, has 160 calories, 3 grams fat, and 28 carbohydrates.

The larger sized tortilla used for burritos, weighs 2–3 ounces and runs as high as 190 calories, 5 grams of fat, and 32 carbohydrates (remember, in each case these numbers represent only *one!*). So, when you get *four* tortillas as a side dish at a Mexican restaurant, that will add up to 640 calories, 12 grams fat, and 112 grams carbohydrates (see Tortilla Wraps, p. 77).

6. Lentils. The lentil is a marvel of both high fiber (15 grams for 1/4 cup) and excellent texture. We keep a pot of cooked lentils to add to our soups and casseroles. It freezes well when cooked (see Lentils, p. 89).

7. Couscous. This is almost the "lightest" of the grains. One cup will fluff up to 3 1/2 cups and serve six people for just 88 calories a serving (18 carbohydrates) when cooked (it only takes 6 minutes). We prefer to cook them in a good stock in order to enhance the flavor (see p. 90).

8. Carbohydrates. Whenever the carbohydrate levels go above 30 grams (after having deducted the fiber, also in grams), then you may want to reduce the "starch" content of the meal. An example is the Indian Ocean Gumbo (p. 135) that has 54 grams net carbohydrate. With 30 grams as a reasonable/moderate goal for diabetics and others trying to lose weight, it is obviously high by 24 grams. The rice is the major starch player, so you can reduce its impact by cutting your 1/2 cup cooked to a 1/4 cup. Always remember the *30-gram limit* and halve the portion of *starch*–it's a good general option.

CULINARY TECHNIQUES

1. Draining Pasta to Perfection. Every pasta sauce should be fully completed before the final act of cooking and draining the pasta. I always drain mine through a stainless steel colander set in a large heatproof bowl. The pasta drains and the boiling water heats the bowl.

I pour off the water (when the bowl is hot) and use this warmed bowl to toss the pasta. In this way, it drains and retains its heat. Please don't keep pasta sitting over the water; it will set up into a solid lukewarm "cake" (see Leaf Greens and Sausage Pasta, p. 71).

2. Tossing Pasta. Pasta, by its very nature, is mostly a light cream color, and unless it's sauced, it is flat, floury, and non-reflective. *Not very appealing!* This is why good oils are added, both for flavor and that glossy light-reflecting finish. Of course, this means added calories from fat, albeit mostly good monounsaturated oils. But there is a limit–and this is often exceeded because it tastes *so* good! I use a reduced stock (often chicken) that compliments the dish, and I thicken this with very little arrowroot (see p. 37, n. 7). The ratio is 1 level teaspoon to 1/2 cup stock. Use this mixture to add that final glisten. The flavors are good and the reflection looks just like a quarter cup of oil (2 ounces oil = 500 fat calories)! (See Pasta with Mushrooms and Peas, p. 75.)

3. Poële. This is rarely listed in basic techniques because it is basically a sauté (shallow fried) that is finished by part poaching and part steaming. It is far and away our favorite vegetable dish, and it is a wonderfully creative base for all kinds of added protein. Please do give it a try. I believe it has the potential for becoming a family favorite (see Poële plus variations, pp. 78, 80).

4. Large Green Leaves. There are several to choose from. The Swiss chard (with the "designer colored stems"—red, yellow, and orange), kale, collards, and mustard greens all have a heavy central stalk that is best stripped from the tender leaves. I roll the leaves into two portion "bundles" and store them in plastic bags for up to seven days. I like to slice them into fine pieces (1/4 inch) and then cut again to shorten each "ribbon." They are then steamed or scattered into casseroles, soups, and stews (see Steamed and Sautéed Green Leaf Vegetables, p. 98).

5. Fresh Vegetable Peelings. Yes, I know, peeling vegetables has now been reduced to the level of Flintstone inconvenience, and yet they are budget worthy contributions to really nourishing meals. We always save the peelings (having washed them thoroughly) in a large plastic freezer bag and then use them when we are making a good stock (see Pan Roasted Root Vegetables, p. 100).

6. Salad Dressings/Tossing. For several years now, we've used an old plastic salad spinner to both rinse and dry our salad leaves and then dress the salad! Just pour on an oil-and-vinegar styled* dressing (it doesn't work well with thick "mayonnaise" dressing), and spin it off. Decant the used dressing into a bottle and keep refrigerated for up to one week—used repeatedly, it should always be used up within that time. You get a perfect salad, evenly coated, and less pools of dressing going to waste (*see Treena's Dressing, p. 84).

7. Thickenings. For my purposes (where fewer calories from refined calories and saturated fats are my goal), I do not use a flour and butter "roux" as a thickening. I prefer to use a "slurry" of cornstarch or arrowroot. A slurry is a mixture of water/stock or wine and the starch, stirred until it is a lump-free cream-like consistency (usually 2 Tablespoons liquid to 1 Tablespoon starch for 1 to 2 cups to be thickened).

The liquid to be thickened is taken off direct heat, the "slurry" is added, and the dish stirred well and then returned to the heat to boil for 30 seconds in the case of cornstarch, in order to remove the taste of "starch." Arrowroot will thicken and clear at just below the boil.

Both of these starches need to be used at the last minute before serving because they thin out quite rapidly (see Tilapia in Coconut Cream Sauce, p. 109).

8. Garlic. For some, garlic is an unacceptable flavor, possibly due to its overuse by an enthusiastic amateur! For such folks, it is possible to use the prebaked whole head of garlic (wrapped in foil and roasted 1 hour). The cooked garlic can be trimmed flat across the top and then the soft center squeezed out as a much less pungent garlic paste (see Halibut Northwestern Style, p. 116).

9. Dry Before Fry. Most "flesh" foods–meat, poultry, fish–are up to 70 percent moisture content. These need to be dabbed dry before shallow-frying or grilling, then seasoned and sometimes sprayed lightly with olive oil. This allows for better, more even, browning, especially when the pan temperature is up to the *needed* 350°F. I always use paper towels for this purpose and rinse my hands afterward (see Chicken Stir-Fry, Thai Style, p. 163).

10. Yogurt Cheese. This is a good idea: it reduces fat and calories and develops good taste. The problem is that it involves *change,* and that is sometimes hard. Your shopping list changes, your preparation changes, and the culinary techniques change–but you can easily save about 70,000 calories a year by changing to this one idea. And at 3,500 calories for one pound of human body fat–that's 20 pounds!

I use Dannon NonFat Plain Yogurt because it has no starch binders (thickeners) added. I buy the 32-ounce container and use a sharp pointed tool (carving fork in my case) to puncture, from the outside in, the empty plastic tub across the base and up the sides for 3 inches. You'll need dozens of small holes for it to work.

I then use a second 32-ounce yogurt and tip it into the "strainer" and place it over a measuring jug to catch the drips of whey as they separate from the curd. I leave the unit (covered with the plastic lid) in the refrigerator for at least 12 hours. You can expect just under 16 ounces of whey to drain into the jug. (I've yet to find an "acceptable" use for the whey, so it's discarded. *Do let me know if and how you use it!*) You now have what can be called "fresh cheese" or "yogurt cheese." It can be combined 50/50 with "I Can't Believe It's Not Butter!®" to reduce fat spread calories, . . . or used in place of sour cream. You can add maple syrup to taste as a sweet "cream" for pies and Jellos. It can also make a great sauce (see Curried Chicken with Sweet Potatoes, p. 173).

11. Yogurt Sauce. The best way to use yogurt as a sauce "combination" is to reduce it to "fresh cheese" as shown in "Yogurt Cheese" above and included in several recipes. For a good example see Chicken a la Keene, p. 171, step 3).

Because yogurt cheese, made from nonfat plain yogurt has, in fact, *no fat,* it does make it easier to curdle if poorly handled.

The ways to avoid this are as follows:

A. Thicken the liquid base (i.e. stock or other thin cooking "broth") with a cornstarch slurry (1 level Tablespoon of cornstarch to 2 Tablespoons water mixed to lump-free "cream" for each 1 cup of thin liquid) and boil for 30 seconds to "cook" the starch.

B. Use 1/3 cup of yogurt cheese for every 1 cup of thickened sauce base.

C. Pour 1/4 cup of hot sauce *only* into the yogurt cheese to *temper* the cheese. This means to warm it up and begin to combine it with the starch used to thicken the sauce's base. Pour this "tempered" cheese back into the rest of the sauce. Keep hot but do not boil.

Using this technique will prevent a curdle and you can try creating your own "cream" sauces with virtually no added fat.

12. Onions and the Initial Sauté. To get the best out of an onion (and garlic) used in stews, soups, and casseroles, it is necessary to "sweat" it in a little oil. By "sweat" I mean to shallow-fry the onion slices (or fine dice) in olive oil (see discussion on light [aroma] oils, etc., p. 29, n. 3) for *at least* five minutes. At the 300°F mark, the oil will rupture the microscopic sacks in the onion and release volatile oils that are not released by simmering or boiling. The cells literally "sweat out" the oils in the extra heat and make a great deal of flavor difference in the finished dish.

How much oil to add? My rule of thumb is 1 teaspoon to each medium onion, or 1 tablespoon for each 1 pound.

In my past I always called for 1/4 cup (2 oz.) of clarified butter for each 1 pound onions. That's more than 400 calories versus 1 tablespoon of olive oil at 119 calories. Not a bad start to create great food with less risk (and less cost)! (See Chicken Curry Sri Lanka Style, p. 138, to show how spices can be added.)

13. Cooking Larger Amounts and Freezing. Now and again pre-prepared and frozen dishes (that exactly match our taste and individual nutritional needs) are a great benefit—as long as it's *now and again.* The convenience is an amazingly powerful motivation that can eventually lead you into a whole arena of manufactured foods that will rob you of essential individuality and creativity.

Any stewed meat and vegetable dish can be treated this way. A good example is the Italian Meat Sauce with Turkey on page 156. It's also a great way to test out the 14 1/2-inch skillet (see p. 41, n. 3).

Here are a couple of hints if you do decide to try it. When the meat sauce (or stew) is done, measure it in 2-person servings (just over 1 cup), put it into good Ziploc® freezer bags, and exhaust the air as you zip it up. Lay it flat and slip it into a sink full of ice cubes and water to cool quickly. Dry the bags and write the name and date. When cooled, lay the bags on a flat metal sheet (cookie pan, etc.) and put them into the freezer. When frozen solid, you can store them upright—zip outward for ease of removal—like a filing system.

We *always* serve our prefrozen meals with lots of fresh vegetables, taking a fraction of the time we saved and truly upgrading the meal's celebration.

14. Velvet Sauces. Like many good ideas, this started as an accident! I had steamed some parsnips until very soft and had put them in a blender with some evaporated skim milk to puree (make smooth-ish). I had just started the blender when the phone rang. The blender whizzed on for 7 minutes (our phone had a depressing meter that "counted"!) I came back to discover *velvet.* The plant cellulose had "moved in with" the milk proteins and became as ultra smooth as an Alfredo sauce. I retested the idea with sweet potatoes and again with peas (you'll need to sieve the sauce to get rid of the stubborn outer "shells"). It works! You can blend for as little as 4–5 minutes, but somehow the magic seems better at 6–7 minutes, providing you can stand the noise! The sauce can be used with pasta and aided with a tablespoon of good grated parmesan sprinkled over the top (remember, the sauce itself is fat free). Look at how it works in Turkey Potpie (p. 158).

15. *Tomato and Wine Sauce for a Sauté (or Baste).* It may seem too nongourmet to use tomato ketchup, but I invite you to try it in the London Broil on page 178. If you like it as much as I do, then try it with chicken drumsticks or with barbecued ribs as a baste—it *works!*

16. *Brown on One Side.* Most domestic pots and pans are quite small and unsuited for the chefs' method (with large pans and the 10,000 BTUs of gas stovetops) of high heat brisk searing and tossing that browns all sides. Meats are about 70 percent moisture, so when the diced meat is added to a hot "small" pan, it's hard to get an all over "browning" before the moisture is driven to the surface and the meat boils or simmers instead.

I use the *one-sided* deep browning made possible with a hot pan and a little oil (1 Tablespoon per 2 to 3 pounds works). I get flavor and color and a somewhat better flavor penetration of the meat itself! I certainly avoid the stewing problem.

17. *The Omelet Party.* This is not so much a technique as an idea for a simple party that's a lot of fun.

Depending upon how many guests your house can hold, it usually works best to have one omelet maker for each twelve guests— and enough elbow room for each to handle the "whisking and folding." Our son Andy and I have done more . . . but that's because he is competitive enough to feed an army!!

You can choose finely cut garnishes and set these out with teaspoons in small dishes for your guests to select their custom filling. Some examples include baby shrimp, sliced black olives, capers, fine-chopped bacon, diced Roma tomato and/or sun dried tomatoes, chopped red onion, roasted garlic paste, grated cheese, chopped roasted red peppers, fine chopped chipotle peppers, parsley, basil, pine nuts—the list is almost endless!

Each guest prints their first name on a small (8 oz.) clear plastic "glass." They fill the glass about half full with fillings (4 oz. is plenty of filling). They then hand their glass to the omelet-maker, who makes the omelet from a bulk mix (see p. 54). We use a ladle that measures the exact amount needed. The happy guest then goes off with their very own omelet and grabs a salad and some crusty bread. That's it—and it's always been a great success!

EQUIPMENT

1. *Steamer.* By far the easiest steamer and least expensive is the expanding stainless steel unit that opens with flower-like metal "petals" to fit most mid-sized saucepans. My only gripe is that their feet/legs are too short. I need 1 1/2 inches of space between the pan base and the steamer and the legs are usually 1/2 to 3/4 inches.

2. *Microwave.* I've come to accept the microwave oven now that it can come complete with convection (fan-driven heated air). The microwave does a good job on Potato Diamonds-in-the-Jacket (p. 103) and is really good at poaching fish (see Tilapia, p. 113).

3. The Wide Skillet. Most skillets simply aren't wide enough or don't have a thick enough base to withstand warping over high heat after many uses over multiple years. I've come to the conclusion that some things should be the best there is because they will last, literally, for a lifetime. The old trusted and true cast-iron cookware will definitely last *if you clean it properly.* A wide skillet, however—up to 12 1/2 inches—is almost too heavy to handle. We found the new "professional" grade Scanpan to be a perfect blend of weight, size, and ease of cleaning. It is, of course, expensive, but judging by its usefulness, it can get more than three hundred uses a year for about 75 cents a use. Try dividing the use times into the cost of a mixing machine or a food processor or a good gas barbecue, and I think you'll find that the simple skillet does well by use/cost comparison.

The largest skillet (in normal domestic distribution) allows for the preparation of eight to ten portions of skillet stews—enough to prepare ahead and freeze for *those* days when nothing seems to go right! (See our Basque-style Skillet Stewed Chicken, p. 161.) And the larger surface area allows you to cook several fish fillets, steaks, or veal escallops without crowding.

4. Pan Temperature. It is now possible to get the right heat for a good sauté (shallow-fry) of about 350°F. There is a small, heavy based barbecue rack thermostat with two loop handles. You simply put it into the skillet as you let the pan heat up before use.

Component Design (NW)
P.O. Box 10947, Portland, OR 97296
1-800-338-5594

5. Vertical Chicken Roaster. There are a large number of variations on this simple "gadget." They all work by being inserted into the "neither regions" of the bird and then set upright in a roasting pan. It works well with a convection oven but because of its height won't fit any microwave I've ever seen (see Hawaiian Curried Chicken, p. 140).

6. Fat Strainer. This is far and away the most important piece of equipment for the caring cook who needs to limit saturated fats. The jug is made of heavy Lexan (heatproof plastic) and has a curious spout that comes from the bottom, rather than the top. This allows the fat to rise to the surface and permits you to pour fat-free juices from under the fat layer (see Coq au Vin, p. 169).

7. Thermometers. There are two essential thermometers you'll need no matter what you cook or for whom.

A. *Meat Thermometer (digital).* This is a thin probe that penetrates meat, fish, or liquids and reads off the "internal" temperature. This is vital to ensure that food temperatures rise to the 165°F needed to kill off practically all known bacteria (see pp. 42–45 for additional safety information).

B. *Refrigerator (free-standing).* This measures and monitors your refrigerator temperature, which *must* be kept at 40°F or below. Above 40°F, harmful bacteria flourish! (Again, *please* see safety notes on the following pages.)

HOME FOOD SAFETY

Background

For several years until 2006, I have had the good fortune to serve on what is called a blue ribbon panel (of "experts") created by the American Dietetic Association (ADA) and ConAgra Foods, the giant food manufacturer's nonprofit foundation that does splendid work for those in need.

I was fortunate because I got to understand the size of this problem and to search for solutions alongside some of the brightest and best scientists of our time.

A great deal can be done to prevent the estimated 24 to 81 million—yes MILLION—cases of "food borne diarrhea disease" that occurs each year in the United States. One estimate of the cost to our economy is $5 to $17 billion—yes BILLION—every year.

The best solution is incredibly simple and highly personal; in fact, it's in YOUR (and my) hands.

Here is the basic plan:
1. Control the amount of bacteria present in food.
2. Prevent what there is from multiplying.
3. Destroying bacteria at correct cooking temperatures.
4. Preventing cross-contamination.

And here is what you and I can do to achieve these goals.

1. Personal Hygiene

We need to wash our hands often and well, especially after every single restroom visit and when handling raw foods.

We need hot running water and "ordinary" soap (in the long term special antibacterial soaps may damage your skin).

We need a good nail brush (keep our nails short) and wash for as long as it takes to sing "Happy Birthday to Me" twice!

I prefer then to use a paper towel to dry them.

2. Correct Temperatures

a. We can keep bacteria counts low by refrigeration—at 40°F and below; above 40°F and the risk goes up degree by degree. Have an internal thermometer in your fridge to be sure.

b. Serve hot food as soon as it is cooked. If you have to keep it hot, be sure it stays above 140°F. (*Note:* This is why a digital thermometer with a probe is essential in every family kitchen.)

c. If you've cooked a larger amount of food, like big casseroles, divide it up into smaller amounts to help it cool quicker.

d. Heat to at least 140°F all bottled and canned, especially home-preserved foods, before tasting them.

e. All cooked foods should exceed 140°F (again it's important to use a probe thermometer, and digital is best.)

f. If there is any doubt . . . throw it out!

3. Kitchen Hygiene

This is mostly about cross contamination. It would seem obvious that the entire kitchen should be kept very clean. All floors, walls, and ceilings as well as countertops are important.

The most frequent source of food poisoning, however, comes from cross contamination in which, for example, raw foods, poultry, game, meats, and so on, come in contact with cooked foods that are then eaten without heating.

I had an especially nasty time with a potato salad at a very good hotel in Chicago that was traced back to exactly that source.

It's important to use separate chopping boards (useful to have a set with different colors). Knives and other implements must also be washed well in hot soapy water before being used for a different task. Counter surfaces can be cleaned with a light spray of chlorinated water and a paper towel (not a cloth towel or sponge).

4. Shopping

Make your food shopping the last thing you do before heading home. Put perishables in foil bags or a cooler and never leave food out of refrigeration for longer than two hours.

When you get plants home (vegetables and fruit) wash them well in cold running water before you put them away (except mushrooms, which spoil when washed ahead of time).

5. Defrosting

Frozen foods can sometimes be defrosted with a microwave, but this can, unfortunately, partly ruin the texture of many foods.

It's always best practice to thaw frozen foods at the 40°F temperature where you will usually need 24-36 hours depending upon the size of the food.

It is extremely unwise to set a package out at room temperature to defrost; remember any temperature between 40°F and 140°F is in a real danger zone.

6. Freezing

If you have made a larger quantity of stew or soup and want to freeze it for later use, I suggest you put it hot into small (2-4 portion) Ziploc styled bags, exhaust the air, and then chill them quickly in a sink of iced water before putting them into the deep freeze.

Summary

I'm extremely grateful for the work done by Al Wagner Jr., who serves with the Texas Agricultural Extension Service. He came up with quite a comprehensive list that covers most of our potential risks in a very brief format. He has kindly allowed me to reproduce it for you.

Please read it through once . . . it will be enough to provide you with the reason why we have 24-81 million cases of food poisoning a year. It doesn't have to happen to you or those you love.

Please see the tables on the next two pages!

BACTERIAL FOOD POISONING CHART

Bacteria Responsible	Description	Habitat	Types of Foods	Symptoms	Cause	Temperature Sensitivity
Staphylococcus aureus	Produces a heat-stable toxin	Nose and throat of 30 to 50 percent of healthy population; also skin and superficial wounds	Meat and seafood salads, sandwich spreads and high salt foods	Nausea, vomiting and diarrhea within 4 to 6 hours; no fever	Poor personal hygiene and subsequent temperature abuse	No growth below 40°F. Bacteria are destroyed by normal cooking but toxin is heat-stable.
Salmonella	Produces an intestinal infection	Intestinal tracts of animals and man	High-protein foods: meat, poultry, fish, and eggs	Diarrhea nausea, chills, vomiting, and fever within 12 to 24 hours	Contamination of ready-to-eat foods, insufficient cooking, and recontamination of cooked foods	No growth below 40°F. Bacteria are destroyed by normal cooking.
Clostridium perfringens	Produces a spore and prefers low oxygen atmosphere. Live cells must be ingested.	Dust, soil, and gastrointestinal tracts of animals and man	Meat and poultry dishes, sauces and gravies	Cramps and diarrhea within 12 to 24 hours; no vomiting or fever	Improper temperature control of hot foods, and recontamination	No growth below 40°F. Bacteria are killed by normal cooking but a heat-stable spore can survive.
Clostridium botulinum	Produces a spore and requires a low oxygen atmosphere. Produces a heat-sensitive toxin.	Soils, plants, marine sediments, and fish	Home-canned foods.	Blurred vision, respiratory distress, and possible DEATH	Improper methods of home-processing foods	Type E and Type B can grow at 38°F. Bacteria destroyed by cooking and the toxin is destroyed by boiling for 5 to 10 minutes. Heat-resistant spore can survive.
Vibrio parahaemolyticus	Requires salt for growth.	Fish and shellfish	Raw and cooked seafood	Diarrhea, cramps, vomiting, headache, and fever within 12 to 24 hours	Recontamination of cooked foods or eating raw seafood	No growth below 40°F. Bacteria killed by normal cooking.
Bacillus cereus	Produces a spore and grows in normal oxygen atmosphere.	Soil, dust, and spices	Starchy food	Mild case of diarrhea and some nausea within 12 to 24 hours	Improper holding and storage temperatures after cooking	No growth below 40°F. Bacteria killed by normal cooking, but heat-resistant spore can survive.

BACTERIAL FOOD POISONING CHART

Bacteria Responsible	Description	Habitat	Types of Foods	Symptoms	Cause	Temperature Sensitivity
Listeria monocytogenes	Survives adverse conditions for long time periods	Soil, vegetation, and water; can survive for long periods in soil and plant materials	Milk, soft cheeses, vegetables fertilized with manure	Mimics meningitis. Immuno-compromised individuals most susceptible	Contaminated raw products.	Grows at refrigeration (38-40°F.) temperatures; may survive minimum pasteurization temperatures (161°F for 15 seconds)
Campylobacter jejuni	Oxygen sensitive, does not grow below 86°F	Animal reservoirs and foods of animal origin	Meat, poultry, milk, and mushrooms	Diarrhea, abdominal cramps, and nausea.	Improper pasteurization or cooking, cross-contamination	Sensitive to drying or freezing; survives in milk and water at 39°F for several weeks
Versinia enterocolitica	Not frequent cause of human infection	Poultry, beef, swine; isolated only in human pathogen	Milk, tofu, and pork	Diarrhea, abdominal pain, vomiting; mimics appendicitis	Improper cooking; cross-contamination	Grows at refrigeration temperatures (35-40°F); sensitive to heat (122°F)
Enteropathogenic E. coli	Can produce toxins that are heat stable and others that are heat-sensitive	Feces of infected humans	Meat and cheeses	Diarrhea, abdominal cramps, no fever	Inadequate cooking; recontamination of cooked product	Organisms can be controlled by heating; can grow at refrigeration temperatures.

Recipes

BREAKFAST
AND BRUNCH

The Patriot...Summer Cereal

SERVES 2

This is now a special treat. The carbs are a challenge for Treena. I simply try not to smack my lips too much!

INGREDIENTS

2 cups	BRAN FLAKES
2 Tablespoons	FRESH MILLED FLAXSEED
1/2 cup	BERRY FRUIT (I like strawberries.)
1/2 cup	BLUEBERRIES (fresh or frozen)
1	BANANA
1/4 cup	SEED NUT MIX (see p. 61)
2 Tablespoons	BROWN SUGAR or Splenda™
1 cup	VANILLA SOYMILK, chilled

BEFORE YOU COOK:

Measure the cereal, Seed Nut Mix, et al. Hull and wash berries. Peel and slice banana.

METHOD OF ASSEMBLY

1. Put bran flakes with flaxseed into bowls.
2. Add fruit and Seed Nut Mix.
3. Sweeten with sugar or Splenda™.
4. Pour on chilled soymilk to taste.

NUTRITIONAL ANALYSIS

Per serving: 538 calories, 14 g protein, 81 g carbohydrates, 22 g fat, 2 g saturated fat, 3% calories from saturated fats, 365 mg sodium, 84 mg calcium, 14 mg iron, 312 RE Vitamin A, 31 mg Vitamin C, 9 mg Vitamin E, 16 g fiber

AT A GLANCE
(FOR SKILLED COOKS IN A HURRY)

Measure bran into bowls. Add seed nut mix and flax seed. Top with washed berries and banana. Sweeten with sugar or Splenda™. Use well-chilled soymilk. Don't forget the word *yum!*

Granola Parfait

Here is another patriotic breakfast idea. I like to think that I started the idea way back in 1978. You can find it today in many of the better hotel chains but made with a somewhat less red, white, and blue emphasis. . . . It is fiddly enough to fix when you have company or as a Mother's Day treat perhaps?

INGREDIENTS

1/2 cup	LOW FAT GRANOLA
1 cup	LOW FAT PLAIN YOGURT
1/2 teaspoon	COCONUT ESSENCE
2 ounces	STRAWBERRIES
2 ounces	BLUEBERRIES
1/2 teaspoon	SPLENDA ™
1/4–1/2 teaspoon	FRESHLY GROUND BLACK PEPPER (optional)

BEFORE YOU ASSEMBLE:

Wash berries briefly. Dry on paper towels. Measure the rest. Dust berries with Splenda ™ and black pepper.

METHOD OF ASSEMBLY

1. Choose a plain glass (8-oz. size, preferably tall and narrow).
2. Alternate layers of berries, yogurt, and granola to get the red, white, and blue appearance.
3. Serve nice and cold. A mint leaf looks great as a garnish!

NUTRITIONAL ANALYSIS

Per serving: 200 calories, 8 g protein, 34 g carbohydrates, 4 g fat, 1 g saturated fat, 5% calories from saturated fats, 148 mg sodium, 242 mg calcium, 1 mg iron, 138 RE Vitamin A, 22 mg Vitamin C, 1 mg Vitamin E, 3 g fiber

Winter Cereal

When the early morning temperature drops to around 50°F, we shift over to our oatmeal breakfast. Even though it takes fifteen minutes, we use that time to shower and dress following our morning walk. The oatmeal has real texture and nuttiness; it seems to stick to our ribs. People who loathed oatmeal as children often love ours as adults.

INGREDIENTS

1 cup	ROLLED OATS (not instant, please)
1/2 cup	SEED NUT MIX (see p. 61)
1/4 cup	RAISINS
2 1/2 cups	LIGHT VANILLA SOYMILK
2 Tablespoons	FRESHLY GROUND FLAXSEEDS
To thin	VANILLA SOYMILK (optional)
1/2 cup	STRAWBERRIES (in season)
1 Tablespoon	BROWN SUGAR or SPLENDA™, or a mix of both

BEFORE YOU COOK:

Measure all ingredients. Hull and wash berries, and slice.

COOKING METHOD

1. Combine oats, seed nut mix, raisins, and soymilk in a small saucepan. Cover and cook on low heat 15 minutes.
2. Stir well. Bring to a boil, stirring constantly for 2 minutes. Add flaxseeds, replace lid, and lower heat.
3. Spoon into warmed bowls, top with berries if you are using them, and sprinkle with your choice of sugar or Splenda™. Serve cold soymilk on the side.

NUTRITIONAL ANALYSIS

Per serving without added soymilk or berries: 484 calories, 14 g protein, 59 g carbohydrates, 24 g fat, 3 g saturated fat, 6% calories from saturated fats, 160 mg sodium, 98 mg calcium, 4 mg iron, 3 RE Vitamin A, 1 mg Vitamin C, 8 mg Vitamin E, 8 g fiber

*Note: Reduce the **volume** by half if you are diabetic or trying to lose weight.*

AT A GLANCE
(FOR SKILLED COOKS IN A HURRY)

Cook oats, seed nut mix, raisins, and soymilk for 15 minutes on low heat—stir to boil. Boil and cover, reduce heat, then add flaxseed. Serve with berries, sugar, and cold soymilk.

Boiled Eggs and "Soldiers" SERVES 1

You must have heard the expression "I can't even boil an egg" as a description of someone who finds it difficult to cook. Actually, boiling water is pretty basic, yet there are some small but clever little wrinkles to getting the perfect boiled egg, whether "just runny" at 4 minutes or usefully hard at 8–10 minutes.

INGREDIENTS

2	LARGE FRESH EGGS (We use Omega-3-fed or free-range.)
1 teaspoon	SALT dissolved in cooking water
1 slice	WHOLE WHEAT TOAST
2 teaspoons	I CAN'T BELIEVE IT'S NOT BUTTER!® (LIGHT)
Season	FRESHLY GROUND SEA SALT
Season	FRESHLY GROUND WHITE PEPPERCORNS

BEFORE YOU COOK:

Bring eggs out of the fridge for about an hour to reach room temperature.

COOKING METHOD

1. Bring water and salt to a boil, then remove from heat. Add the eggs gently, lowering them in with a spoon.
2. Return pan to heat and use an oven or digital timer to count 4 minutes from the moment the water boils.
3. At minute 4, remove eggs with a slotted spoon to a bowl and serve *immediately.* If you have an unavoidable delay, you can crack the sharp end of the shell to release some of the pent-up heat and slow down the overcooking process caused by containment.
4. *The Soldiers.* This is the term used by us former (and current) "Brits." We "butter" the toast and then cut it into fingers (like a line of soldiers). Treena and I then season the buttered top lightly with salt and white pepper. Treena taps her egg top (now sitting upright in either an egg cup or a napkin ring) and picks off the broken shell. I, being who I like to think I am, take a swipe at the top/side (half an inch down) with a serrated blade knife and swiftly saw my way across. It's your choice! We eat a little with a small egg spoon and then dip away with the "seasoned" soldiers.
5. *Hard-boiled.* Exactly the same lead-up but allow 8–10 minutes for medium to extra large eggs. Then, leave them in the saucepan and run cold water over them for a minute. Drain all liquid and "rustle" the eggs hard enough to gently crack the entire shell surface. Refill the saucepan with cold water and begin to peel the eggs *under* the water, they *will* slip off easily (they do for me!). They can then be cooled and used as you will.

NUTRITIONAL ANALYSIS

Per serving: 310 calories, 16 g protein, 25 g carbohydrates, 17 g fat, 4 g saturated fat, 12% calories from saturated fats, 927 mg sodium, 71 mg calcium, 3 mg iron, 258 RE Vitamin A, 0 mg Vitamin C, 2 mg Vitamin E, 3 g fiber

Scrambled Eggs (Egg Beaters Method)

Whole eggs are splendid food—convenient, quick to cook, and a reasonably priced excellent source of protein. However, they all add up (over time) with saturated fat, cholesterol, and therefore calories. We save our whole eggs for boiled in the shell and poached (although both now need to be well cooked). At other times we scramble a yolk-free mix called Egg Beaters™, but it needs special handling to work really well.

INGREDIENTS

1/2 teaspoon	NONAROMATIC OLIVE OIL
1/2 cup	EGG BEATERS™ (plain)
1/4 teaspoon	HERBS OF PROVENCE (dried)
season	SALT and WHITE PEPPER

BEFORE YOU COOK:

Measure all ingredients. Combine eggs, herbs, and seasonings.

COOKING METHOD

1. Heat small nonstick skillet, add oil, and warm over medium-high heat.
2. Pour the egg mixture directly into the pan. Leave for 1 minute without stirring.
3. Using a flat-ended spatula, pull the sides into the middle all the way round, heaping the moist folds in the center.
4. Turn the piled eggs over quickly to just heat, about 10 seconds. It must be moist. Turn out and serve.

NUTRITIONAL ANALYSIS

Per serving: 80 calories, 12 g protein, 2 g carbohydrates, 2 g fat, 0 g saturated fat, 0% calories from saturated fats, 780 mg sodium, 40 mg calcium, 2 mg iron, 120 RE Vitamin A, 0 mg Vitamin C, 3 mg Vitamin E, 0 g fiber

AT A GLANCE
(FOR SKILLED COOKS IN A HURRY)

Combine egg with seasonings and herbs. Heat small pan. Add oil and heat med/high. Pour in and leave 1 minute. Draw sides to center all round and heap in center. Turn over to warm surface (10 seconds). Serve.

Scrambled Eggs (Regular Eggs)

*Here is our whole egg method for those who simply **must** have the added mouth feel of fat **occasionally**. This is not a daily "fix." It's an occasional way of having non-runny eggs (see p. 51).*

INGREDIENTS

1/2 teaspoon	NONAROMATIC OLIVE OIL or BUTTER
2 large	EGGS (We use Omega-3-fed or free-range.)
2 Tablespoons	NONFAT HALF & HALF
season	SALT and WHITE PEPPER

BEFORE YOU COOK:

Break eggs into bowl, beat lightly, and add seasonings. Measure cream.

COOKING METHOD

1. Heat a small skillet on medium and add oil or butter. If you are using butter, wait until it just begins to brown.
2. Pour in the seasoned eggs, stirring gently as it sets.
3. When it's almost completely set, pour in the cold, fat-free half and half and stir back up to heat. *Note: The cold cream stops the eggs from overcooking.*

NUTRITIONAL ANALYSIS:

Per serving: 189 calories, 13 g protein, 4 g carbohydrates, 12 g fat, 3 g saturated fat, 14% calories from saturated fats, 732 mg sodium, 49 mg calcium, 1 mg iron, 191 RE Vitamin A, 0 mg Vitamin C, 2 mg Vitamin E, 0 g fiber

AT A GLANCE
(FOR SKILLED COOKS IN A HURRY)

Mix eggs with seasoning. Heat oil or butter in pan. Add eggs and stir to cook. Add cream when just done. Serve.

Whole Egg Omelet with Mushrooms and Bacon

Occasionally we bust loose and have a special omelet. This happens as a brunch and sometimes as a party idea. (See p. 40, n. 17, for "The Omelet Party.") We don't recognize the U.S. family-styled restaurant omelet as an omelet; it's more like griddled, rolled up, and scrambled. See ours below and compare!

INGREDIENTS

4 large	WHOLE EGGS (preferably Omega-3-fed)
2 Tablespoons	NONFAT HALF AND HALF
1/4 teaspoon	SALT
1/4 teaspoon	WHITE PEPPER

Filling:

spray	NONAROMATIC OLIVE OIL (spray)
2 slices	CANADIAN BACON
4	WHITE MUSHROOMS (1-inch diameter)
1/4 teaspoon	DILL WEED
1/4 teaspoon	SALT
1 teaspoon	DRIED WILD MUSHROOM POWDER (optional) (see Buying: p. 31, n. 13)

BEFORE YOU COOK:

Break eggs. Bring to room temperature. Measure rest of ingredients. Finely slice the Canadian bacon and cut mushrooms in quarters, including the stems. Use a 7-inch nonstick omelet pan.

COOKING METHOD

1. Mix the eggs with the half and half and seasonings. Beat lightly.
2. Heat the Canadian bacon in a pan sprayed with oil.
3. When the bacon sizzles, add mushrooms. Dust with dill, wild mushroom powder, and salt. Stir-fry for 2 minutes. Turn out on a plate to keep warm.
4. To cook the eggs: Heat the omelet pan over medium-high heat. Spray with olive oil. When it begins to smoke, add egg mixture.
5. Shake the pan back and forth and mix with a figure-eight motion with a large fork until they are almost done but still moist on the surface.

6. Spread the warm filling down the center at right angles to the handle. Fold the handle side over the filling with a spatula and push across the pan to fold the other side over.
7. Grip the handle underneath with your right hand palm facing up. Hold a warm plate in your left hand and turn the omelet out by bringing your right hand up and over the plate. (Now you see why we need television!)
8. I like to spray the top of the omelet with a little oil to make it glisten.

Note: Please see how you can use this idea for a party. It's great fun for everyone! *(See p. 40.)*

NUTRITIONAL ANALYSIS

Per serving: 196 calories, 16 g protein, 3 g carbohydrates, 13 g fat, 4 g saturated fat, 18% calories from saturated fats, 914 mg sodium, 51 mg calcium, 2 mg iron, 191 RE Vitamin A, 0 mg Vitamin C, 2 mg Vitamin E, 0 g fiber

AT A GLANCE
(FOR SKILLED COOKS IN A HURRY)

Combine eggs with half and half. Season. Sauté Canadian bacon with mushrooms and dill (add wild mushroom powder–optional). Make omelet. Fill with mushrooms. Serve.

Sauté Sausage and Tomatoes

This is one of our all-time favorites for a change of scene at breakfast. Our best bet for sausages are those made with chicken that is carefully seasoned (about 7 grams of fat per 86-gram link). Turkey sausages are improving, but others are simply too high in fat to fit our lifestyle. In any case, when split and stuffed with tomato, the lower fat factor simply melts away. Do always check the sodium if you have hypertension—they all tend to be high.

INGREDIENTS

1 teaspoon	OLIVE OIL SPRAY
2 3-ounce	LOW FAT, LOW SODIUM ITALIAN TURKEY SAUSAGES
2	MEDIUM TOMATOES
season	SALT and WHITE PEPPER
1/4 teaspoon	HERBS OF PROVENCE

BEFORE YOU COOK:

Core the tomatoes and cut in half. Season with salt, pepper, and herbs.

COOKING METHOD

1. Heat a small nonstick skillet and spray with oil. Add sausages, turning in the oil to coat, and brown over medium-high heat.
2. Using tongs, keep turning to color evenly, 5 minutes.
3. Lower the heat to medium and add tomatoes, round side down. Cover and cook for 5 minutes.
4. Turn the tomatoes over and turn the sausages to a less browned side. Cover and cook for the last 5 minutes.
5. To serve, split the sausage down the center lengthways. Leave a hinge at the bottom. Fill the sausage with one half of a tomato, crushed. Set the other half on the side.

NUTRITIONAL ANALYSIS

Per serving: 251 calories, 12 g protein, 15 g carbohydrates, 5 g fat, 1 g saturated fat, 4% calories from saturated fats, 1,010 mg sodium, 36 mg calcium, 2 mg iron, 76 RE Vitamin A, 27 mg Vitamin C, 1 mg Vitamin E, 1 g fiber

AT A GLANCE
(FOR SKILLED COOKS IN A HURRY)

Heat skillet and mist with oil. Add sausage to brown evenly 5 minutes. Add seasoned tomato halves. Cover and cook for 5 minutes. Lower heat, turn tomatoes/sausage and simmer. Split sausage and stuff with 1/2 tomato, placing other half on side.

Pancakes—Extra Thin

MAKES 9 PANCAKES (SERVES 4)

*Chat with anyone with a British background and mention pancakes (in the extra-thin crêpes style) and see their eyes sparkle! The best known are served with a scattering of sugar and freshly squeezed lemons. Our Norwegian neighbors love them rolled around lingon berries with sour cream and, of course, sugar. But a universal favorite is the lemon. Thick pancakes, like those served in the U.S., are called "dropped scones," "pikelets," or "griddle-cakes." The huge breakfast stack served at a typical, American commercial breakfast is an excellent example of commercialization, in which we, the consumer, are supposed to feel that we've got our money's worth. But then how much does it cost to lose the weight? Try these pancakes as a **treat** solution–perhaps your eyes could sparkle too?*

INGREDIENTS

1	WHOLE LARGE EGG
1	EGG YOLK
1 cup	2% MILK
1/2 teaspoon	VANILLA EXTRACT
1/2 cup	ALL-PURPOSE FLOUR
1 teaspoon	NONAROMATIC OLIVE OIL
1 teaspoon	BROWN SUGAR
1 teaspoon	SPLENDA™
1	LEMON

BEFORE YOU COOK:

Separate the second egg for the yolk. Measure the remaining ingredients. Quarter the lemon.

COOKING METHOD

1. Beat the whole egg, egg yolk, milk, and vanilla in a bowl. Whisk in the flour. Let mixture rest for 30 minutes before cooking. (The starch cells break down and produce a finer, less-starchy result.) Combine the brown sugar and Splenda™.
2. Warm a shallow sided 7–8 inch nonstick fry pan over medium heat. Add the oil. Swish it over the pan and then tip the oil into the batter and whisk it in.
3. Measure 1/4 cup of batter into skillet and gently roll it around the pan to evenly coat the surface. When the top becomes dull and waxy (takes 30–50 seconds), just lift one edge with a spatula. Hold this edge lightly and slide the spatula under the whole width. Now, lift it up and turn it over. (You'll get the idea after a couple. That's why there's enough for nine!)
4. Cook the other side for about 15–20 seconds and slide out of the pan onto a stack. Cover with a napkin.

5. There is enough fat in the eggs to make the batter nonstick. No need to add more oil.

6. The best serving method is to turn them out onto hot plates directly from the pan. Sprinkle with the sugar mix and serve with the lemon—and watch them sparkle!

NUTRITIONAL ANALYSIS

Per serving: 139 calories, 6 g protein, 17 g carbohydrates, 5 g fat, 2 g saturated fat, 13% calories from saturated fats, 49 mg sodium, 93 mg calcium, 1 mg iron, 86 RE Vitamin A, 6 mg Vitamin C, 1 mg Vitamin E, 0 g fiber

AT A GLANCE
(FOR SKILLED COOKS IN A HURRY)

Combine eggs, milk, and vanilla. Whisk in flour. Let rest for 30 minutes (the batter, not you!). Heat crêpe pan. Add oil, coat pan, and then tip remaining oil into batter. Make crêpes. Serve with sugar mix and lemon.

Black Tea

*Okay, I admit it; one of the first recipes turns out to be **tea!** For years I've tried to convince people in North America (especially in the U.S.) to bring the water up to the boil and **not** use 170–180°F water sitting ready for use on coffee heaters! So here is our method. Try it; you may be surprised!*

INGREDIENTS

4 cups	WATER (filtered to reduce chlorination)
2 bags	BLACK TEA (I like Tetley's English Breakfast.)
1/4 cup	2% MILK

BEFORE YOU COOK:

Measure ingredients, and preheat (using hot water or microwave) the teapot.

COOKING METHOD

1. Bring filtered water up to the boil.
2. Pour out the prewarming water in the teapot, if used.
3. Add the tea bags, pour in just-boiling water, and stir twice.
4. Cover and wrap teapot in a "cozy" (insulated cover).
5. Allow to steep for 4 to 5 minutes.
6. Put about 2 Tablespoons cold milk into a cup, add tea, and stir.

Optional: Sugar, Splenda™, or honey can be added to sweeten.
Fresh lemon slice can be used instead of milk.

NUTRITIONAL ANALYSIS

Per serving: 15 calories, 1 g protein, 1 g carbohydrates, .5 g fat, 0 g saturated fat, 0% calories from saturated fats, 15 mg sodium, 37 mg calcium, 0 mg iron, 17 RE Vitamin A, 0 mg Vitamin C, 0 mg Vitamin E, 0 g fiber

AT A GLANCE
(FOR SKILLED COOKS IN A HURRY)

Warm teapot. Bring filtered water up to boil. Add water to bags, cover, and steep 4 to 5 minutes. Serve with milk or lemon. Use sugar, Splenda™, or honey as sweetener.

Hot Chai Tea

Our midmorning breaks have become as important as afternoon tea. (For a Brit, that is quite an admission!) Our favorite hot beverage is Chai, which is a gently spiced sweet tea to which we add vanilla soymilk. The choice of 2% milk or soy is yours.

INGREDIENTS

4 teaspoons	POWDERED CHAI	1 cup	BOILING WATER
1 cup	VANILLA SOYMILK		

BEFORE YOU COOK: Measure all.

COOKING METHOD

1. Combine Chai mix with milk. Pour in the boiling water. Mix well.
2. Reheat in the microwave for 1 to 2 minutes.

Iced Chai

Here is our warm-weather midmorning drink, the one we have for a break with our fruit duo (see p. 85). Check to be sure your blender is designed to crush ice, and give it enough time to do the job.

INGREDIENTS

4 teaspoons	CHAI TEA POWDER
2 cups	VANILLA SOYMILK
1 cup	ICE CUBES (to fill one 12-oz. serving glass)

COOKING METHOD

1. Mix chai powder with soymilk.
2. Pour into blender. Add one glass of ice cubes.
3. Blend about 2 minutes to fully crush the ice.
4. Let stand for 5 minutes; then stir well and serve with a straw.

NUTRITIONAL ANALYSIS

Per serving: 120 calories, 3 g protein, 21 g carbohydrates, 2.5 g fat, .5 g saturated fat, 1% calories from saturated fats, 120 mg sodium, 20 mg calcium, 0 mg iron, 0 RE Vitamin A, 0 mg Vitamin C, 0 mg Vitamin E, 0 g fiber

Seed Nut Mix

*If you threw your breakfast cereal out of the window into your garden (or window box) would it come up as a plant? More than likely **not!***

*Ours would because we use a **small** handful of raw mixed nuts and seeds to garnish and add texture to our processed cereals. Each seed and some nuts have the amazing ability to sprout and, when properly tended, to grow. They present an excellent food source with both good fats and protein. Consume too many and it poses a calorie problem, but a small handful each and every day will make an excellent contribution to your future health.*

Wherever possible, buy from bulk because they are lower in cost and usually fresher. Keep the seeds and nuts in a cool, dry, airtight container. Buy enough to use up completely every 3 to 4 weeks.

The eventual "mix" is up to you and your preferences. Here are the ones we use.

INGREDIENTS

Nuts

8 ounces	ALMONDS, chipped or fine sliced
8 ounces	WALNUTS SMALL (broken) PIECES
8 ounces	PECANS FINELY CHOPPED (expensive)
8 ounces	HAZELNUTS (you chop finely)

Seeds

8 ounces	SUNFLOWER
8 ounces	PUMPKIN

The above mix will produce 3 pounds, or 50 servings, that usually lasts us for one month. I don't mix in ground flax seeds, but add them separately to our cereal (1 Tbsp. per person per day).

NUTRITIONAL ANALYSIS

Per serving: 166 calories, 5 g protein, 5 g carbohydrates, 16 g fat, 2 g saturated fat, 11% calories from saturated fats, 1 mg sodium, 32 mg calcium, 2 mg iron, 3 RE Vitamin A, 5 mg Vitamin C, 7 mg Vitamin E, 2 g fiber

Recipes

LUNCHES
OR SUPPERS

Tactful Soup

We love the idea of "getting to our food fast before someone gets there first." Because of this we almost always buy and use fresh food. Now and again, however, we upgrade the humble can of soup. After trying them all, we've settled on the Progresso brand for flavor and content (even though the sodium is too high). We add simple flavors and colors and always enjoy the result. It makes an ideal supper after a long day's drive.

INGREDIENTS

1	CLOVE GARLIC, crushed
1 teaspoon	FINELY CHOPPED GINGER ROOT
1 teaspoon	OLIVE OIL
16-ounce	CANNED SOUP (see Buying, p. 29, n. 1)
1 cup	FROZEN MIXED VEGETABLES (frozen peas, beans, corn, carrots)
Optional	
1/4-pound	COLD ROASTED MEAT

BEFORE YOU COOK:

Crush and chop the garlic. Grate or fine chop the ginger. Open the soup, measure the vegetables, and dice the meat into 1/4-inch pieces.

COOKING METHOD

1. Heat a medium-size saucepan over medium heat.
2. Add the oil with the ginger and garlic. Stir 2 minutes.
3. Add the soup, frozen vegetables, and meat, if you are using it. Cover and bring to the boil slowly. Cook 5 minutes.

NUTRITIONAL ANALYSIS

Per serving with chicken breast: 299 calories, 28 g protein, 29 g carbohydrates, 7 g fat, 1 g saturated fat, 3% calories from saturated fats, 828 mg sodium, 67 mg calcium, 5 mg iron, 421 RE Vitamin A, 3 mg Vitamin C, 1 mg Vitamin E, 9 g fiber

FABIS
(The Cream of Soups)

*Many years ago, while serving as the general manager of the Royal Ascot Hotel, I created what we then called the Farmhouse Vegetable Soup with Cream. It was very popular! Since then I've continuously upgraded this idea (see FABIS on p. 35). Here is the best to date, but that isn't the end of it. There's always **yours** from where you live—or visit?*

INGREDIENTS

1 Tablespoon	OLIVE OIL
2 cups	CHOPPED YELLOW ONION
1 large clove	GARLIC, crushed
1 teaspoon	SALT
1 1/2 pounds	SWEET POTATOES, roughly chopped
1 1/2 pounds	CARROTS, roughly chopped
1 Tablespoon	HERBS OF PROVENCE
2 1/2 cups	LOW-SODIUM VEGETABLE STOCK (see p. 222)
1 cup	PLAIN SOYMILK
Optional	
1/4 cup	FAT-FREE HALF AND HALF
garnish	CHOPPED PARSLEY

BEFORE YOU COOK:

Wash all vegetables and drain dry. Roughly chop onion, carrots, sweet potato. Crush garlic. Measure the remaining ingredients.

COOKING METHOD

1. Heat a medium-size saucepan on medium heat. Add oil.
2. Add onions and fry for 10 minutes to color.
3. Add the garlic and fry for 1 minute. Stir in the carrots, sweet potatoes, and herbs. Season with salt and fry together for 10 minutes.
4. Pour in vegetable stock and bring to a boil. Cover and cook at a slow boil for 30 minutes.
5. Purée in a blender, adding the plain soymilk. Season to taste with salt and pepper. Garnish with chopped parsley and serve half and half on the side if you are using it. Each cup has 3 to 4 servings of vegetables!

NUTRITIONAL ANALYSIS

Per serving: 231 calories, 6 g protein, 46 g carbohydrates, 3 g fat, 0 g saturated fat, 0% calories from saturated fats, 487 mg sodium, 82 mg calcium, 2 mg iron, 5676 RE Vitamin A, 44 mg Vitamin C, 2 mg Vitamin E, 8 g fiber

AT A GLANCE
(FOR SKILLED COOKS IN A HURRY)

Wash vegetables; peel and chop roughly. Crush garlic. In medium saucepan, heat oil and sauté onions 10 minutes. Add garlic, stir, and add carrots and sweet potato. Sauté 10 minutes. Add stock, herbs, salt and boil 30 minutes. Blend until smooth. Add soymilk. Serve half and half on the side.

Tomato Soup with an Italian Twist

SERVES 4

I'm going to assume that you and your family like tomato soup. (If not, then skip this page!) Having got used to the standard canned version, you may be approaching boredom—or at least **silent acceptance!**

In just a couple of extra minutes you can brighten things up a bit by following an Italian method. Served with a good roasted vegetable bread (p. 104), it makes a great supper.

INGREDIENTS

1 teaspoon	OLIVE OIL
1/2 cup	SWEET ONION, finely chopped
1 clove	GARLIC
1 teaspoon	BASIL, dried
1 teaspoon	OREGANO, dried . . . (or Northwest Italy Ethmix™)
2 cups	DICED TOMATOES, canned
1 1/2 cups	FILTERED WATER (see p. 29, n. 2)
1/2 teaspoon	SALT (only if tomatoes are unsalted)

BEFORE YOU COOK:

Finely chop onion, crush the garlic, and measure the remaining ingredients.

COOKING METHOD

1. Heat the oil in a saucepan. Add the onion, garlic, and herbs and sauté 5 minutes.
2. Add the tomatoes, water, and salt (if necessary). Bring to the boil, then reduce to simmer for 10 to 15 minutes. It's ready!

NUTRITIONAL ANALYSIS

Per serving: 40 calories, 1 g protein, 6 g carbohydrates, 1 g fat, 0 g saturated fat, 0% calories from saturated fats, 390 mg sodium, 76 mg calcium, 0 mg iron, 14 RE Vitamin A, 19 mg Vitamin C, 0 mg Vitamin E, 1 g fiber

Minestrone

Surely everyone knows this great soup, one that changes with both season and region. It has more meat in the poorer south of Italy and more vegetables in the richer north. This is typical of the north. If served with some good roasted vegetable bread (p. 104) and a salad, it makes a perfectly sustaining family dinner.

INGREDIENTS

Basil Pesto

2 Tablespoons	CHOPPED FRESH BASIL LEAVES
2 Tablespoons	PINE NUTS
1 clove	GARLIC
1 Tablespoon	PECORINO ROMANO CHEESE

Soup

1 teaspoon	NONAROMATIC OLIVE OIL
1	MEDIUM ONION
3	RIBS CELERY
4	CARROTS
1/2 pound	RED POTATOES
7 cups	HOT WATER
1 1/2 teaspoon	SALT
1/4 pound	SMALL SHELL PASTA
1 (15-oz. can)	CANNELLINI or other white beans
1 pound	ROMA TOMATOES (or 1 14.5-oz. can diced tomatoes in juice)
1 bunch	SPINACH
1 teaspoon	EXTRA VIRGIN OLIVE OIL
6 Tablespoons	GRATED PECORINO ROMANO CHEESE
6	LEAVES OF FRESH BASIL

BEFORE YOU COOK:

Crush garlic, chop basil, chop the onion, celery, carrots, red potatoes, and tomatoes into 1/2 inch pieces. Drain and rinse the canned beans. Wash and stem spinach, then cut to 1/4-inch x 1-inch pieces. Finely slice basil for garnish. Measure the remaining ingredients.

COOKING METHOD

1. Place the basil, pine nuts, garlic, and cheese in a small processor and whiz to a paste. Scrape into a small bowl, spray the top with olive oil and lay a small piece of plastic wrap directly on top of the pesto to keep it from turning black.
2. Heat the oil in a high-sided skillet or small Dutch oven. Sauté the onion on medium high until it starts to get soft, about 2 minutes. Add the celery, carrots, and potatoes and continue cooking 3 minutes. Pour in the hot water; cover and bring to a boil. Stir in the salt and pasta and boil, uncovered, 6 minutes.
3. Add the pesto, beans, tomatoes, spinach, and extra-virgin olive oil. Bring back to a boil and it's ready to serve. Sprinkle grated cheese and chopped basil on each serving.

NUTRITIONAL ANALYSIS

Per serving: 287 calories, 46 g carbohydrate, 7 g fat, 2 g saturated fat, 6% calories from saturated fat, 818 mg sodium, 9 g dietary fiber

AT A GLANCE
(FOR SKILLED COOKS IN A HURRY)

Process the parsley, basil, olive oil, nuts, garlic, and cheese to paste (Pesto). Heat oil in saucepan. Sauté onion. Add celery, carrots, and potatoes (3–5 mins.). Add hot water; cover and boil. Stir in salt and pasta—boil uncovered for 6 minutes. Add Pesto, beans, tomato, spinach, and oil. Return to serving temperature. Garnish with cheese and fresh basil.

Parsley Pesto

If fresh basil is hard to find, try this fresh parsley pesto made with dried basil.

2 Tablespoons chopped fresh parsley	2 Tablespoons pine nuts or walnuts
1 Tablespoon dried basil	1 clove garlic, bashed and chopped
1/8 teaspoon extra-virgin olive oil	1 Tablespoon grated Pecorino Romano cheese

Combine parsley, basil, olive oil, nuts, garlic, and cheese in a small processor and whiz to a paste.

Spinach Salad with Pineapple and Avocado

SERVES 2

*We have many salads, and really enjoy the variety and quantity of both fruit and vegetables that we get at each tossing. Here is just one example of a **greens**-based combination. There is enough for two of us as a main dish.*

INGREDIENTS

4 cups	BABY SPINACH LEAVES
1/4 pound	BABY BOK CHOY
1/4 pound	CELERY HEART
6 ounces	FRESH PINEAPPLE
1 small	AVOCADO
2 Tablespoons	TREENA'S DRESSING (p. 84)

BEFORE YOU COOK:

Wash everything well. Dry spinach leaves gently, and slice the bok choy every 1/2 inch. Separate leaves. Cut celery same size. Dice pineapple and avocado, and mix to prevent browning.

COOKING METHOD

1. Combine all ingredients in a large bowl and keep very cold until just before serving.
2. Add dressing and toss well. Serve immediately.

NUTRITIONAL ANALYSIS

Per serving: 228 calories, 5 g protein, 15 g carbohydrates, 18 g fat, 2 g saturated fat, 8% calories from saturated fats, 216 mg sodium, 154 mg calcium, 7 mg iron, 541 RE Vitamin A, 65 mg Vitamin C, 3 mg Vitamin E, 12 g fiber

Composed "Fruited" Salad

*There are two **basic** styles of salad. The "tossed" with its ingredients well mingled (see p. 69) and the "composed" where each food is separate yet artfully presented. This is one of those.*

INGREDIENTS

8 ounces	ICEBERG HEAD LETTUCE
2 large leaves	ROMAINE GREEN LETTUCE
4	RADISH
8	BLACK GRAPES (seedless)
1/4	ROCK MELON (cantaloupe)
2 large	STRAWBERRIES (in season)
2 Tablespoons	TREENA'S DRESSING
Optional	
2 crackers	PUMPKIN CHEESE FLATBREAD (see Buying, p. 34, n. 32)
drizzle	EXTRA-VIRGIN OLIVE OIL

BEFORE YOU COOK:

Cut iceberg into 2 wedges (4 oz. each). Select good green leaves of romaine (wash well and dry). Cut radish, strawberries, and grapes in half. Slice melon; remove seeds and skin. Serve as one piece.

COOKING METHOD

1. Lay the deep green leaf on a dinner plate. Place the wedge of iceberg on plate left, then the melon slice. Cluster the grapes, strawberry, and radish to plate right.
2. Serve the pumpkin cheese flatbread on extreme plate right.
3. Serve the dressing on the side—along with extra-virgin olive oil to drizzle more or less at will!

Leaf Greens and Sausage over Pasta

I love the robust flavors in this dish, and the serving sizes are perfect for me. For Treena, I usually reduce the pasta to 1 ounce (raw), 1/4 cup cooked, and add 1/2 cup of shallow fried fennel bulb (or celery). This deals with the extra carbs that trouble some of us—and it tastes great!

INGREDIENTS

1/2 pound	DRY WHOLE WHEAT SPAGHETTI (see note above)
1 teaspoon	OLIVE OIL
1 cup	CHOPPED ONION
2 cloves	GARLIC, bashed and chopped
2	LOW-FAT CHICKEN ITALIAN SAUSAGES
1/4 teaspoon	FENNEL SEEDS
8 cups	MUSTARD GREENS (2 bunches of leaves) or 2 packages frozen
1/4 teaspoon	SALT
1/4 teaspoon	PEPPER
1 Tablespoon	BALSAMIC VINEGAR
1/2 teaspoon	CRUSHED RED PEPPER
2 Tablespoons	GRATED PARMESAN CHEESE

BEFORE YOU COOK:

Chop the onion and crush the garlic. Cut sausage into 1/2-inch slices. Wash and slice the mustard greens. Measure the rest.

COOKING METHOD

1. Cook the spaghetti according to package directions. Drain and keep warm in a colander over a bowl of hot water.
2. Heat the oil in a high-sided skillet on medium high. Sauté the onion 2 minutes or until it begins to turn translucent. Add the garlic and cook 1 more minute. Toss in the sausage and fennel seeds and cook 2 minutes or until lightly browned on the outside.
3. Stir in the mustard greens, cover, and cook on low until they wilt but are still bright green—about 5 minutes. Toss with the spaghetti and season with salt, pepper, balsamic vinegar, and red pepper. Serve when heated through with Parmesan cheese sprinkled over the top.

NUTRITIONAL ANALYSIS

Per serving: 349 calories, 53 g carbohydrate, 5 g fat, 1 g saturated fat, 3% calories from saturated fat, 202 mg sodium, 6 g dietary fiber

AT A GLANCE
(FOR SKILLED COOKS IN A HURRY)

Cook pasta *al dente* (slightly undercooked). Heat oil, sauté onion, and then add garlic. Add sliced sausage and fennel seeds. Cook 2 minutes to brown. Stir in greens; cover and cook on low to wilt (5 mins.). Toss in pasta. Season with salt, pepper, balsamic vinegar, and red pepper. Serve hot with dusting Parmesan.

Spaghetti Carbonara

*I get just a **little** "miffed" about the Americanization of this wonderful Italian classic. Apparently someone decided to add a cream sauce that not only ruins the original "taste" but makes it over-rich. I'll admit that mine is the absolute opposite and also "different" from the Italian carbonara (bacon and eggs over pasta with grated cheese). I added taste, aroma, color, and texture . . . not just a blanket of white!*

INGREDIENTS

8 ounces	UNCOOKED SPAGHETTI
1 teaspoon	SALT
1/2 teaspoon	NONAROMATIC OLIVE OIL
3 ounces	CANADIAN BACON
2 Tablespoons	PINE NUTS
4	SUN-DRIED TOMATO HALVES
1/2 cup	EGG SUBSTITUTE
2 Tablespoons	CHOPPED PARSLEY
2 Tablespoons	CHOPPED CHIVES, or 1 finely chopped green onion
1/4 teaspoon	FRESHLY GROUND BLACK PEPPER
1/8 teaspoon	SALT
1/4 cup	GRATED PARMESAN CHEESE

BEFORE YOU COOK:

Cut bacon into 1-inch "match sticks." Cut sun-dried tomatoes into thin strips. Measure the remaining ingredients.

COOKING METHOD

1. Bring a large pan of water to a boil and drop in the spaghetti and salt. Stir and cook for 10 minutes once it comes back to the boil.
2. While you wait for the spaghetti to cook, heat the oil in a medium-sized skillet and add the Canadian bacon, pine nuts, and sun-dried tomatoes. Fry—stirring—until the pine nuts are golden and the bacon is lightly browned. Set aside.
3. Set a colander over a large heatproof bowl. Pour the spaghetti (water and all) into the colander. Take the colander out of the water and set on a plate to drain. Pour the hot water out of the bowl. Now the bowl is hot enough to finish the dish.
4. Tip the spaghetti into the hot bowl. Add the bacon mixture, egg substitute, parsley, chives, pepper, salt, and cheese. Toss to mix and watch as the hot pasta cooks the egg substitute. Serve immediately on preheated plates with a dusting of Parmesan.

NUTRITIONAL ANALYSIS

Per serving: 324 calories, 46 g carbohydrate, 8 g fat, 2 g saturated fat, 5% calories from saturated fat, 526 mg sodium, 2 g dietary fiber

AT A GLANCE
(FOR SKILLED COOKS IN A HURRY)

Boil water for pasta. Cook spaghetti 10 minutes (*al dente*). During this time, heat skillet. Add oil. Sauté bacon, dried tomatoes, and pine nuts together until light brown. Set aside. Put colander over heat-proof bowl. Pour just-cooked spaghetti and water into colander (the water will heat the bowl). Throw out water, and turn drained pasta into hot bowl. Add sautéed bacon mix and the eggs, parsley, chives, and cheese. Toss well to mix and "cook" the eggs. Serve *immediately*.

Pasta with Mushrooms and Peas

As a swift, simple supper dish, this is hard to beat. The portion size may seem small when compared to the twelve to sixteen ounces of pasta typically served in some well-meaning restaurants, but then those rack up as many as a thousand calories. That's okay as an occasional treat, but surely not for a reasonable supper at home. If carbs concern you, just halve the pasta and double the mushrooms.

INGREDIENTS

1/2 pound	DRY BUTTERFLY (or another shape you like) PASTA
1 teaspoon	NONAROMATIC OLIVE OIL
1/2 cup	CHOPPED ONIONS
1/4 pound	LEAN SMOKY HAM
1/2 pound	CREMINI OR WHITE BUTTON MUSHROOMS
2 cups	PETIT PEAS
1/4 teaspoon	SALT
1/4 teaspoon	PEPPER
1 teaspoon	ARROWROOT or cornstarch
1/2 cup	CHICKEN BROTH
1/4 cup	GRATED PARMESAN CHEESE

BEFORE YOU COOK:

Cook pasta according to package directions. Chop the onions. Cut ham in 1/4-inch pieces. Quarter the mushrooms. Thaw the peas.

COOKING METHOD

1. Cook the pasta according to package directions. Drain and keep warm in a covered colander over hot water.
2. While the pasta is cooking, heat the oil in a high-sided skillet on medium-high. Cook the onion, without browning, until it starts to wilt and turn translucent. Stir in the ham and mushrooms, and cook until the mushrooms are done, about 5 minutes.
3. Add the peas and reserved pasta and cook, stirring, just until heated through. Season with salt and pepper. Combine the arrowroot with the broth and pour into the hot pasta. Stir until it thickens and gets glossy. Divide among four hot plates, sprinkle with Parmesan, and serve with a nice green salad.

NUTRITIONAL ANALYSIS

Per serving: 379 calories, 59 g carbohydrate, 6 g fat, 2 g saturated fat, 5% calories from saturated fat, 720 mg sodium, 7 g dietary fiber

AT A GLANCE
(FOR SKILLED COOKS IN A HURRY)

Cook the pasta, and hold in colander over hot water. While pasta cooks, heat oil, sauté
onion, and add ham and mushrooms. Toss together until mushrooms are *just* cooked.
Add peas with pasta. Stir to heat through. Thicken broth. Pour over pasta. Sprinkle with
cheese.

Roast Beef Toaster Tortilla Wraps

SERVES 1

*Cold roast beef is **not** a cheap leftover— it actually costs as much as ten dollars a pound! So we treat it with great respect—as a **treat**. Using the small 5-inch diameter flour tortillas, we make up our own toaster tortilla wraps. They are fun, fast, and can be stored in the deep freeze as an emergency snack.*

INGREDIENTS

1	FRESH TORTILLA
1 ounce	GOAT CHEESE
1 Tablespoon	HORSERADISH
2 ounces	COLD ROAST BEEF (round rump roast)
1 ounce	NONFAT PROVOLONE CHEESE (Alpine Lace brand)
1 to 2 ounces	ROASTED RED PEPPERS, bottled or homemade
6 leaves	FRESH CILANTRO

BEFORE YOU COOK:

Measure all ingredients. Combine goat cheese with horseradish. Finely shred the roast beef (makes it easier to eat). Combine shredded beef, roasted peppers, and cilantro.

COOKING METHOD

1. Spread the tortilla with the goat cheese/horseradish mixture. Top with the provolone slice.
2. Add the beef/red pepper/cilantro mixture.
3. Fold in half and press down firmly to seal. If you are making more than one, you can now wrap each as a single in a sandwich bag and store in a freezer-quality zip-top bag in the freezer.
4. To cook, put folded side down into a toaster set on maximum brown. It may need a second heating of a little less time if frozen.

NUTRITIONAL ANALYSIS

Per serving: 390 calories, 32 g protein, 27 g carbohydrates, 17 g fat, 9 g saturated fat, 21% calories from saturated fats, 733 mg sodium, 249 mg calcium, 3 mg iron, 261 RE Vitamin A, 1 mg Vitamin C, 1 mg Vitamin E, 1 g fiber

AT A GLANCE
(FOR SKILLED COOKS IN A HURRY)

Spread 5-inch tortilla with goat cheese/horseradish mixture. Add Provolone slice and shredded roast beef/roasted pepper/cilantro mixture. Seal and heat in toaster.

The Perfect Poële (Basic Method)

SERVES 4

In the winter months when root vegetables abound, we have our favorite poële dishes. A poële is a mixture of diced root vegetables shallow-fried with garlic and ginger and then finished in a stock. All manner of proteins can be added, the stocks changed to suit, and special seasonings added. You can double the recipe and freeze the extra for that sudden need for a meal in a moment.

INGREDIENTS

1 Tablespoon	OLIVE OIL
1 cup	SWEET ONION, sliced thin
1 clove	GARLIC, crushed
1 Tablespoon	CHOPPED GINGERROOT
1 cup	PARSNIP, cut 1-inch pieces
1 cup	TURNIP, cut 1-inch pieces
1 cup	RUTABAGA, cut 1-inch pieces
1 1/4 cups	CARROT, cut 1-inch pieces
1 1/4 cups	CELERY, cut 1-inch pieces
1 Tablespoon	HERBS OF PROVENCE
1 teaspoon (max.)	SALT
2 cups	VEGETABLE STOCK (see p. 222)
1 Tablespoon	CORNSTARCH

BEFORE YOU COOK:

Wash all vegetables, drain, and peel. (Keep all the peelings for stock.) Cut into even-sized cubes—about 1/2 to 1 inch. Measure the herbs. Finely slice (toothpick size) the ginger. Crush the garlic.

COOKING METHOD

1. Heat a large skillet on medium high. Heat the oil and sauté onion 5 minutes. Add garlic and ginger and cook another 2 minutes.
2. Now add the carrots, turnips, and rutabagas. Mix well and spread out. Cover and cook 5 minutes to color.
3. Finally add the parsnip, celery, and herbs. Mix, cover, and cook 5 more minutes.
4. Season with 1/4 teaspoon of the salt (add more if you need it, but the herbs and flavors should suffice). Pour in the vegetable stock and bring to a boil. Mix the cornstarch with a little water and add to the stew. Boil 30 seconds to thicken and clear.
5. To serve, add grated Parmesan if you like.

NUTRITIONAL ANALYSIS

Per serving: 130 calories, 3 g protein, 22 g carbohydrates, 4 g fat, .5 g saturated fat, 691 mg sodium, 79 mg calcium, 1 mg iron, 1027 RE Vitamin A, 31 mg Vitamin C, 1 mg Vitamin E, 6 g fiber

AT A GLANCE
(FOR SKILLED COOKS IN A HURRY)

Wash vegetables and peel (reserve for stock), and dice into 1/2-1 inch pieces. Sauté onion 5 minutes. Add garlic/ginger and cook 2 minutes. Add carrot, turnip, rutabaga and stir; cook (covered) 5 minutes. Add herbs, parsnips, celery; cook (covered) 5 minutes. Add stock and herbs; boil till thickened and clear. Taste–correct. Serve.

Poële
(Variations on a Theme) SERVES 4

*Here are some of our variations on a theme using the perfect poële (sauté and steam) idea on page 78. In each case the additions are made at step 4—except for the jellies, which you serve on the side. This is where **your** individual creativity can really shine!*

INGREDIENTS

Roast Duck Poële

1/2 pound	BONELESS DUCK MEAT
1 Tablespoon	LEMON JUICE
2 cups	DUCK STOCK (p. 224)
2 Tablespoons	RED CURRANT JELLY

NUTRITIONAL ANALYSIS

Per serving: 271 calories, 17 g protein, 29 g carbohydrates, 10 g fat, 3 g saturated fat, 294 mg sodium, 87 mg calcium, 3 mg iron, 1040 RE Vitamin A, 33 mg Vitamin C, 2 mg Vitamin E, 6 g fiber

Roast Beef Poële

1/2 pound	ROAST ROUND RUMP (diced 1/2-inch)
4 Tablespoons	HORSERADISH
2 cups	BEEF STOCK (p. 226)

NUTRITIONAL ANALYSIS

Per serving: 276 calories, 21 g protein, 29 g carbohydrates, 12 g fat, 4 g saturated fat, 339 mg sodium, 98 mg calcium, 2 mg iron, 1054 RE Vitamin A, 31 mg Vitamin C, 2 mg Vitamin E, 6 g fiber

Tofu Poële

3/4 pound	FIRM TOFU (1/2-inch cubes)
4 Tablespoons	SOY SAUCE
2 cups	VEGETABLE STOCK (p. 222)

NUTRITIONAL ANALYSIS

Per serving: 187 calories, 10 g protein, 25 g carbohydrates, 6 g fat, 1 g saturated fat, 792 mg sodium, 108 mg calcium, 2 mg iron, 1027 RE Vitamin A, 31 mg Vitamin C, 1 mg Vitamin E, 6 g fiber

Roast Chicken Poële

1/2 pound	ROAST CHICKEN DARK MEAT
1/4 pound	CANADIAN BACON
2 cups	CHICKEN STOCK (p. 225)

NUTRITIONAL ANALYSIS

Per serving 290 calories, 25 g protein, 23 g carbohydrates, 11 g fat, 3 g saturated fat, 707 mg sodium, 90 mg calcium, 2 mg iron, 1039 RE Vitamin A, 31 mg Vitamin C, 2 mg Vitamin E, 6 g fiber

Roast Lamb Poële

1/2 pound	ROAST LEG LAMB MEAT, diced
to taste	LEMON JUICE
2 cups	LAMB OR DUCK STOCK
2 Tablespoons	MINT JELLY

NUTRITIONAL ANALYSIS

Per serving: 273 calories, 19 g protein, 29 g carbohydrates, 9 g fat, 2 g saturated fat, 298 mg sodium, 84 mg calcium, 2 mg iron, 1027 RE Vitamin A, 33 mg Vitamin C, 1 mg Vitamin E, 6 g fiber

Roasted Vegetable Lasagna

*The very broad-noodle pasta pie is one of the most famous Italian dishes. As you can expect, **everyone** has a different favorite way of fixing it, but some people add more meat, more cheese, and more pasta until it becomes more of a threat than a treat. We needed to get it back to normal, so we went for a vegetarian style with roasted vegetables that we love. Try adding your favorite vegetables. This is really good eating!*

INGREDIENTS

Pasta

2 ounces	WHOLE WHEAT LASAGNA, cooked according to package directions (I like Westbrae brand.)

Sauce (for entire recipe)

1/2 teaspoon	NONAROMATIC OLIVE OIL
1 cup	ONIONS, chopped
2 cloves	GARLIC, bashed and chopped
1/2 teaspoon	DRIED BASIL
1/2 teaspoon	DRIED OREGANO
1/2 cup	DE-ALCOHOLIZED RED WINE
1 can	TOMATO PUREE (10 1/2 oz.)
1/8 teaspoon	SALT
1/8 teaspoon	PEPPER

Filling

1/2 cup	LOW-FAT RICOTTA CHEESE
1 Tablespoon	GRATED PARMESAN CHEESE
2 Tablespoons	FRESH BASIL, chopped
1/8 teaspoon	SALT
1/8 teaspoon	PEPPER

Vegetables

1 small	EGGPLANT, cut in 1/2-inch slices
3	ROMA TOMATOES, halved, cored, seeded
8	SHIITAKE MUSHROOMS, stems removed
4 cups	FRESH SPINACH, stemmed and lightly steamed

Topping

2 slices	NONFAT MOZZARELLA CHEESE
1 Tablespoon	PARMESAN CHEESE, grated
1 Tablespoon	FRESH BASIL, chopped

BEFORE YOU COOK:

Cook the pasta and cool. Cut eggplant into 1/2-inch thick slices. Halve, core, and seed tomatoes. Remove stems from shiitakes. Crush garlic and chop herbs. Measure the remaining ingredients.

COOKING METHOD

1. Preheat the oven to 450°F. Heat the oil in a chef's pan on medium. Sauté the onions with the basil and oregano until soft, 5 minutes. Add the garlic and cook 1 minute more. Pour in the wine, tomato puree, salt, and pepper and bring to a boil. Cover and simmer until you are ready to use it but not more than 15 minutes.
2. Lay the eggplant slices, tomato halves skin-side up, and shiitakes on a greased baking sheet with sides. You might need 2 pans. Spray lightly with olive oil pan spray and sprinkle lightly with salt and pepper. Roast 20 minutes in the preheated oven. Set aside. Reduce the oven heat to 375°F. Press the water out of the steamed spinach.
3. Combine the ricotta, Parmesan, salt, pepper, and basil in a bowl.
4. Spoon enough sauce into the bottom of a chef's pan or baking dish to cover thinly. Lay eggplant slices in the bottom of the pan and cover them with another thin layer of sauce. Make a layer of mushrooms and cover with the steamed spinach. Lay the slices of nonfat cheese on top of the spinach. Cover with more sauce, then the ricotta filling. Lay tomatoes over the filling and spread with more sauce. Layer in the noodles. Cover with the remaining sauce.
5. Bake in the preheated oven until heated through (160°F). Because of the density of the dish, this may take as long as 20 minutes. When the sauce is bubbling around the sides, it's hot. Let set for at least 10 minutes before cutting to serve. Combine the Parmesan cheese and chopped basil, and sprinkle over the top.

NUTRITIONAL ANALYSIS

Per serving: 236 calories, 6 g protein, 37 g carbohydrates, 4 g fat, 1 g saturated fat, 4% calories from saturated fat, 747 mg sodium, 325 g calcium, 4 g iron, 356 RE Vitamin A, 37 mg Vitamin C, 3 mg Vitamin E, 10 g dietary fiber

AT A GLANCE
(FOR SKILLED COOKS IN A HURRY)

Heat oven to 450°F. Heat oil. Sauté onions and herbs. Add garlic (additional 1 min. sauté). Add wine, tomato puree, and seasonings. Simmer, covered, up to 15 minutes. Lay vegetables on greased baking sheet(s); spray with oil; season; roast 20 minutes. Combine ricotta, Parmesan, salt, pepper, and basil. Layer the prepared ingredients starting with a little sauce, vegetables, filling, sauce. Top with noodles and sauce. Bake at 375°F for 20 minutes. Stand 10 minutes to set. Dust with cheese and basil.

Treena's Oil and Vinegar Salad Dressing

Throughout the more than fifty years we've shared together, Treena has insisted on her own salad dressing and like her, it's always improving. So here's her latest. I've grown to like it too!

INGREDIENTS

1 Tablespoon	SLICED FRESH GINGERROOT
2 cloves	GARLIC, crushed
1/2 cup	EXTRA-VIRGIN OLIVE OIL
1 cup	TARRAGON WINE VINEGAR
2 teaspoons	LIQUID HONEY
1/2 teaspoon	SALT
1/4 teaspoon	WHITE PEPPER

BEFORE YOU COOK:

Measure all ingredients.

COOKING METHOD

1. Combine all the ingredients in a blender until lump free.
2. Strain through fine sieve into a clean jar with a screw-on lid.
3. Keep refrigerated. Shake well before serving. We use 1 Tablespoon for a single portion of salad.

NUTRITIONAL ANALYSIS

Per serving: 46 calories, 0 g protein, 1 g carbohydrates, 5 g fat, 1 g saturated fat, 20% calories from saturated fats, 47 mg sodium, 1 mg calcium, 0 mg iron, 0 RE Vitamin A, 0 mg Vitamin C, 1 mg Vitamin E, 0 g fiber

Sliced Fruit Duo
(The 11 a.m. Snack)

*The idea behind this page is to look at the 11 a.m. snack as a great way to increase consumption of fruit, turning it into a real (creative?) pleasure and to avoid the cookie, candy, or soft drink "break" that adds calories and **almost** nothing else (plus, **they cost more!**).*

To come up with our list of duos, we first bought almost all the fresh fruit available at our market. We then peeled, sliced (where necessary), and cut each into roughly half-inch cubes. We put each in its own glass or dish.

*We then munch away, putting one fruit with just one other. We were not in complete agreement (what husband and wife ever are!), but in general we did agree. Sometimes it was a **wow;** others were simply pleasant combinations. All our eventual choices were acceptable to us both.*

From this list we were able to create a wide variety of snacks to be served in a small glass with a fork at our midmorning break. It is something we really look forward to every day. A half-cup portion is one fruit serving.

Now it's your turn. Here are our best duos—what about yours?

INGREDIENTS

Primary Fruit	add → Duo 1	or →	Duo 2	or →	Your Duo
MANGO	+ BANANA		+ PINEAPPLE		
KIWI	+ BANANA		+ STRAWBERRY		
ORANGE	+ MANGO		+ KIWI		
GRAPEFRUIT (pink)	+ PEAR		+ ORANGE		
PINEAPPLE	+ APPLE		+ PEAR		
STRAWBERRY	+ KIWI		+ POMEGRANATE		
POMEGRANATE	+ MANGO		+ BANANA		
GRAPES	+ PEAR		+ MANGO		
CHERRIES	+ KIWI		+ PEAR		
APPLES	+ ORANGE		+ GRAPES		
PEAR	+ KIWI		+ PINEAPPLE		
BANANA	+ PINEAPPLE		+ POMEGRANATE		

Recipes

VEGETABLES
AND WHOLE GRAINS

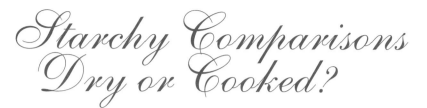

Starchy Comparisons Dry or Cooked?

FOOD	STYLE	DRY QUANTITY	CALS	CARBS	FIBER	PROTEIN	MINUTES TO COOK	NUTRIENTS
Brown Rice	Long Grain	1/4 cup (46 g)	171	36 g	2 g	4 g	35–45	Iron, Thiamine, Niacin, Folate
Wild Rice	Wild	1/4 cup (40 g)	143	30 g	2 g	6 g	45	Vitamin A, iron
Long Grain Rice	Enriched	1/4 cup (46 g)	169	37 g	0 g	3 g	15–20	Thiamine, Iron, Niacin, Folic
Red Beans & Rice	Mix	2 Tbsp (57 g)	180	40 g	5 g	7 g	25–30	Calcium, Thiamin, Iron, Niacin, Folic, Riboflavin
Quinoa	Seed 100%	1/4 cup (43 g)	159	30 g	3 g	6 g	10–15	Iron, Phosphorus, Riboflavin
Couscous	Whole Wheat	1/4 cup (55 g)	210	45 g	7 g	8 g	5–6	Calcium, Iron
Penne Pasta	Soy "flour"	1/2 cup (50 g)	180	15 g	7 g	24 g	12–14	Calcium, Iron
Potato Gnocchi	(pack)	1 cup (204 g)	419	84 g	4 g	13 g	3–4	Iron
Barley	(pearled)	1/4 cup (50 g)	176	39 g	5 g	8 g	45–50	Iron, Thiamin, Riboflavin, Niacin, Phosphorus

COMMENTS ON VARIETY

When considering variety, the need for starch is less compelling than it is for fruit and vegetables. Grains, as you can see from the above list, have a somewhat similar mineral content that makes them (as a group) valuable, but none is a stand-out that demands attention. Yet even though some are relatively weak in some minerals, they are not at the level of empty. So what does one do when selecting for a power pantry?

Here is our list of recommended selections and our reasons why.

1. Brown Rice (long grain). Net carbohydrate (carb minus fiber) is 32 grams. It has a good mineral profile. It is chewy, flavorsome, and sustaining. We cook more than we need and freeze it in 1-cup plastic bags. (See p. 93 for recipe.)
2. Barley. Net carbohydrate is 31 grams. It has a good mineral profile, and it is so good in stews with its wonderful texture. "Pearl" cooks quicker, but it lacks texture/nutrition. (See p. 91 for recipe.)
3. Quinoa. Net carbohydrate is 24 grams. It has good mineral content and is a completely different style of garnish. (See p. 92 for recipe.)

NOTES

1. Wholegrain spaghetti. Though not as attractive as white pasta, it is good for variety and ethnic Italian recipes (see p. 95).
2. Soy "flour" pasta. Net carbohydrate is 8 grams. It doesn't cook as well as white flour pasta and its texture is truly awful!

Fingerling Potatoes

*Treena's diabetes doesn't respond well to plain potatoes, so we have been quietly pleased with a slightly better response to **fingerlings** (perhaps because we eat them skin and all). They are nonetheless delicious, with a pleasant waxy, dense texture. We serve no more than two to three per serving.*

INGREDIENTS

6 ounces	FINGERLING POTATOES (see Buying: p. 31, n. 16)
1/4 teaspoon	SALT
spray	OLIVE OIL spray
2 teaspoons	FINELY CHOPPED PARSLEY

BEFORE YOU COOK:

Wash thoroughly, scrubbing if necessary, but don't peel.

COOKING METHODS

Boiling

1. Bring enough water to cover the potatoes by 1 inch to a boil in a medium saucepan. Add salt.
2. Add fingerlings to the boiling water, cover, and cook for 25 minutes or until just tender.
3. Drain. Spray lightly with olive oil and toss with parsley.

Roasting

1. Add to the roasting pan 30 minutes before the roast is ready to remove from the oven.
2. Add parsley and toss well. No need to add oil.

NUTRITIONAL ANALYSIS

Per serving: 74 calories, 2 g protein, 17 g carbohydrates, 0 g fat, 0 g saturated fat, 0% calories from saturated fats, 284 mg sodium, 9 mg calcium, 1 mg iron, 7 RE Vitamin A, 12 mg Vitamin C, 0 mg Vitamin E, 1 g fiber

Lentils in a Cumin-Flavored Broth

SERVES 4

We really love lentils and have ever since our first visit to India. Dahl is a deeply seasoned lentil dish served as often as rice or beans in the Mexican traditions. It's important to use a good stock at a slow simmer and to catch them when just done—before they begin to "mush." They are helpful for folks with diabetes because their high fiber content slows down the conversion to sugar.

INGREDIENTS

1 1/2 cups	VEGETABLE STOCK (see p. 222) or water
1 cup	LENTILS (green, brown, or red)
1 teaspoon	GROUND CUMIN

BEFORE YOU COOK:

Wash lentils well. Spread out to dry. Discard broken, discolored pieces. Measure remaining ingredients.

COOKING METHOD

1. Bring the stock (or water) to a boil.
2. Rain in the lentils and reduce to a simmer. Cover and cook 30 minutes.
3. Add the cumin in the last 10 minutes. The lentils should be just right after 40 minutes.
4. Taste and add salt only if really necessary!

NUTRITIONAL ANALYSIS

Per serving: 169 calories, 14 g protein, 28 g carbohydrates, .5 g fat, 0 g saturated fat, mg sodium, 33 mg calcium, 4 mg iron, 6 RE Vitamin A, 3 mg Vitamin C, 0 mg Vitamin E, 15 g fiber

Couscous
North African Durum Semolina "Grains"

This classic starch consists of dry, fluffy, tiny grains and is made in less than 6 minutes. It does a fine job of soaking up gravy and can also form the base of an excellent light starch salad. It is usually cooked in water, but I greatly prefer vegetable stock (see p. 222).

INGREDIENTS

1 3/4 cups	VEGETABLE STOCK (or water)
1 cup	COUSCOUS
1 teaspoon	SALT (only if water is used)

COOKING METHOD

1. Heat the vegetable stock in a small saucepan. When it boils, add the couscous and stir four or five times.
2. Remove from heat, cover, and allow to "plump up" for 5 minutes.
3. With a fork, tease the mix to separate the grains.

Note: One cup dry will make 3 1/2 cups of cooked couscous. We use 1/2 cup of lightly packed couscous for a side dish, and a full cup for a salad base.

NUTRITIONAL ANALYSIS

Per 1/2-cup serving: 99 calories, 3 g protein, 20 g carbohydrates, 0 g fat, 0 g saturated fat, 328 mg sodium, 6 mg calcium, 0 mg iron, 0 RE Vitamin A, 0 mg Vitamin C, 0 mg Vitamin E, 1 g fiber

Barley— The Added "Textural" Value

MAKES 12 PORTIONS

If you are someone who has followed my work (and profound changes) over the years, you will know the acronym TACT means **taste, aroma, color, and texture,** *the basic elements of food* **pleasure.** *Texture is last but* **not** *least. In fact, the reason why fats are so well liked is because of their texture or sense of* **mouth roundfulness.** *So texture is vital! I use pot barley, not the more refined* **pearl** *barley to add texture, especially to ground meat dishes where one third of the original meat can be replaced by an equal amount of barley. I brew up a batch of the recipe below and keep it frozen in 1-cup portions. It also works wonders with soups that can do with more "body."*

INGREDIENTS

2 teaspoons	OLIVE OIL
2	LEEKS
4 cloves	GARLIC
3 cups	POT BARLEY
6 cups	FILTERED WATER
1 teaspoon	SALT

BEFORE YOU COOK:

Wash leeks very well, finely slice, then chop. Crush the garlic. Rinse the barley and drain. Measure remaining ingredients.

COOKING METHOD

1. Heat the oil in a saucepan and sauté the leeks with the garlic for 5 minutes.
2. Rinse the barley in a strainer and stir in. Add the water and salt and bring to the boil. Reduce to simmer and cover. Cook for 45 minutes (30 mins. for pearl barley).

NUTRITIONAL ANALYSIS

Per serving: 117 calories, 4 g protein, 23 g carbohydrates, 1 g fat, 0 g saturated fat, 144 mg sodium, 14 mg calcium, 1 mg iron, 1 RE Vitamin A, 1 mg Vitamin C, 0 mg Vitamin E, 5 g fiber

Quinoa ("keen-wa")

This seed-grain is a very attractive starch alternative to the standard potato, pasta, and rice dishes. It also provides an excellent base for a "combined" salad. The grain has been cultivated in South America for more than five thousand years. (See p. 87 for food values and comparisons to other starches.)

INGREDIENTS

2 cups	WATER
1/4 teaspoon	SALT
1 cup	QUINOA
1 Tablespoon	PARSLEY OR CILANTRO, chopped
Optional	
2 teaspoons	WILD MUSHROOM POWDER (see p. 31, n. 13)

BEFORE YOU COOK:

Measure all.

COOKING METHOD

1. Bring water and salt to a boil. Add quinoa all at once. Stir once to get the seeds off the bottom of the pan.
2. When it reboils, turn down to low, cover, and cook for 14 minutes. It will absorb all the liquid.
3. Stir in the parsley or cilantro. We use our powdered wild mushrooms for flavor.

Note: The seed-grain quadruples in size, so one serving is 1 cup cooked. We find that a half cup is plenty, and it's only 83 calories! You can freeze the extra in a zip-top bag for later use.

NUTRITIONAL ANALYSIS

Per serving: 106 calories, 4 g protein, 20 g carbohydrates, 2 g fat, 0 g saturated fat, 99 mg sodium, 18 mg calcium, 3 mg iron, 3 RE Vitamin A, 1 mg Vitamin C, 0 mg Vitamin E, 2 g fiber

Brown Rice (Boil 'n' Steam)

SERVES 4 X 3/4 CUP

I (Graham) have never been a great fan of brown rice. It seemed so stodgy and broken by overcooking. Then we found this long grain brown rice, used my old boil 'n' steam method for the long grain converted rice, and it worked well. It does take twice the time, though, so we always make double and freeze the unused portion. Brown rice is more easily digested by diabetics who need to slow down the conversion to sugars.

INGREDIENTS

5 cups	FILTERED WATER
1/2 teaspoon	SALT
1 cup	LONG GRAIN BROWN RICE

BEFORE YOU COOK:

Put rice in a strainer/sieve and wash well under running cold water.

COOKING METHOD

1. Heat the water in a covered medium-size saucepan.
2. Add the salt. When it boils, add the washed rice.
3. Slow boil the rice in the covered pan for 30 minutes.
4. Turn into a hand sieve and set over rapidly boiling water, tightly covered for another 8 to 10 minutes.
5. You can freeze the cooked rice for future need-it-now moments!

NUTRITIONAL ANALYSIS

Per serving: 171 calories, 4 g protein, 36 g carbohydrates, 1 g fat, 0 g saturated fat, 306 mg sodium, 11 mg calcium, 1 mg iron, 0 RE Vitamin A, 0 mg Vitamin C, 0 mg Vitamin E, 2 g fiber

AT A GLANCE
(FOR SKILLED COOKS IN A HURRY)

Rinse rice well. Pour into boiling salted water (1 c. to 5 c.). Slow boil 30 minutes. Then steam for 8–10 minutes. Can be frozen.

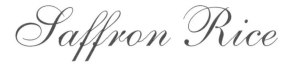

Saffron Rice

SERVES 6

This is a fine, fragrant rice that I can imagine working in a number of different menus. Perhaps it will become a signature dish for you.

INGREDIENTS

1/2 teaspoon	LIGHT OLIVE OIL
3/4 cup	ONION, chopped
1 cup	WHITE RICE, long grain
1 3/4 cups	LOW-SODIUM FISH OR VEGETABLE STOCK (pp. 222–23)
1/4 teaspoon	SALT
1 pinch	POWDERED SAFFRON

COOKING METHOD

1. Warm the oil in a saucepan over medium-high heat. Sauté the onion until translucent, 2 or 3 minutes. Add the rice and cook until it turns chalky white, another 2 or 3 minutes.
2. Pour in the stock and season with the salt and saffron. (*Vegetarian Option:* use vegetable stock.) Cover, bring to a boil, then reduce the heat as low as possible. Cook for 20 minutes, remove from the heat, and set aside for 5 minutes before serving.

NUTRITIONAL ANALYSIS

Per serving: 126 calories, 1 g fat, 0 g saturated fat, 0% of calories from saturated fat, 26 g carbohydrates, 1 g dietary fiber, 3 g protein, 113 mg sodium, 3 RE Vitamin A, 1 mg Vitamin C, 1 mg Vitamin E, 16 mg calcium, 1 mg iron.

Note: This is close to reasonable/moderate at the upper end of the scale and, therefore, needs to be matched to other very low carbohydrate choices on the same plate.

Pasta Angel Hair (Whole Wheat)

*There are of course many different shapes of pasta, and each usually has its correct cooking time printed on the carton—correct for **al dente** (to suit the tooth). Interestingly, the firmer the better, since it takes longer to digest with less adverse impact on our blood sugars. I've grown to prefer the **well-made** whole-wheat variety over the more traditional refined white durum semolina wheat. This basic cooking method is also useful when you want to cook ahead.*

INGREDIENTS

8 cups	WATER
1/2 teaspoon	SALT
4 ounces	WHOLE WHEAT ANGEL HAIR PASTA
1 teaspoon	EXTRA-VIRGIN OLIVE OIL

Optional

2 Tablespoons BASIL, finely sliced

2 Tablespoons PARMESAN, freshly grated

BEFORE YOU COOK:

Measure all. Grate Parmesan if using.

COOKING METHOD

1. Bring the water and salt to a vigorous boil in a medium-large saucepan.
2. Gently push the hard strands of pasta into the boiling water as they soften. Allow to boil for one minute, and be sure each strand is separate. Tongs work well for this.
3. Continue to boil for 6 to 8 minutes (check the package instructions). Subtract 2 minutes if cooking ahead of serving time.
4. Drain the undercooked pasta in a metal colander. Turn into an open ceramic or glass bowl. Drizzle with very little olive oil and toss in the basil. Let cool until needed. Reheat by steaming or tossing with a little extra olive oil in a hot pan. See page 36, note 2, for finishing ideas.

NUTRITIONAL ANALYSIS

Per serving: 253 calories, 12 g protein, 39 g carbohydrates, 6 g fat, 1 g saturated fat, 703 mg sodium, 86 mg calcium, 0 mg iron, 13 RE Vitamin A, 0 mg Vitamin C, 0 mg Vitamin E, 8 g fiber

AT A GLANCE
(FOR SKILLED COOKS IN A HURRY)

Boil water with salt. Add pasta. Cook 6–8 minutes, and drain. If cooking ahead, add oil and basil (optional). Cool. Reheat by steaming, or sauté in olive oil.

Mushrooms on the Wild Side

One of my (Graham's) pet peeves is when restaurants list 'wild' mushrooms and serve the cultivated brown-skinned crimini! I appreciate the expense of fresh wild mushrooms, but they don't taste the same—that is, unless you use this technique (see Buying section and "Before you cook" below).

INGREDIENTS

1 Tablespoon	OLIVE OIL
1/2 pound	CULTIVATED MUSHROOMS, even-sized
1 teaspoon	LEMON JUICE
1/2 teaspoon	SALT
1 teaspoon	WILD MUSHROOM POWDER (see below)

BEFORE YOU COOK:

Find source for supply of dried mushrooms (Frieda's does a good selection). Get 1/2 ounce each of oyster, morel, and shitake (1 1/2 oz. total). Process or pound them into a fine powder. Store in an airtight jar. Cut fresh mushroom into quarters, stalk and all.

COOKING METHOD

1. Wipe mushrooms with a damp paper towel before cutting.
2. Heat medium skillet on medium-high heat (250°F). Add the oil to heat. Toss in the mushroom quarters. Sprinkle with lemon juice, salt, and wild mushroom powder.
3. Stir rapidly to coat evenly for no more than 2 minutes. Serve as a side garnish or incorporate into a stew, casserole, or omelet just before serving.

NUTRITIONAL ANALYSIS

Per serving: 57 calories, 2 g protein, 4 g carbohydrates, 4 g fat, 1 g saturated fat, 282 mg sodium, 2 mg calcium, 1 mg iron, 0 RE Vitamin A, 1 mg Vitamin C, 1 mg Vitamin E, 1 g fiber

AT A GLANCE
(FOR SKILLED COOKS IN A HURRY)

Wipe mushrooms, cut into quarters, and heat oil. Add mushrooms and sprinkle lemon juice, salt, and mushroom powder. Toss and stir 2 minutes max. Serve.

Steamed Summer Squash (Yellow Crookneck)

Summer squash are now available all year, but because they must travel long distances to northern zones in the winter, seasonally they remain best in the summer. Zucchini, Patty Pan, and Crookneck are amongst the best known, with Delicata bridging the gap between summer and winter. We used a 12-ounce yellow crookneck for this recipe, but the one method serves all.

INGREDIENTS

12 ounces	YELLOW CROOKNECK SUMMER SQUASH
season	SALT
season	WHITE PEPPER
1/2 teaspoon	DILL WEED
garnish	PAPRIKA

BEFORE YOU COOK:

Slice the squash in half lengthwise.

COOKING METHOD

1. Bring water in the steamer to a boil.
2. Season the squash with salt, pepper, and dill weed.
3. Lower into steamer to cook for 8 minutes. Test for doneness.
4. Dust with a little paprika for color, and serve.

NUTRITIONAL ANALYSIS

Per serving: 33 calories, 2 g protein, 7 g carbohydrates, 0 g fat, 0 g saturated fat, 306 mg sodium, 41 mg calcium, 1 mg iron, 59 RE Vitamin A, 14 mg Vitamin C, 0 mg Vitamin E, 3 g fiber

AT A GLANCE
(FOR SKILLED COOKS IN A HURRY)

Wash squash—split in two lengthways. Season salt, pepper, and dill weed. Steam 8 minutes. Test for doneness and dust with paprika.

Steamed and Sautéed Green Leaf Vegetables

SERVES 4

Many stores are now doing a much better job stocking green leaf vegetables (other than spinach). Kale, collards, turnip greens, Swiss chard (in designer stalk colors) and mustard greens are examples. We've used Swiss chard as an example of the steam/sauté method.

INGREDIENTS

1 pound	SWISS CHARD (you choose stalk color)
season	SALT
season	WHITE PEPPER
2 teaspoons	OLIVE OIL
2 cloves	GARLIC, fine chopped (optional)

BEFORE YOU COOK:

Wash greens well under running water. Shake dry and strip leaves from stalks (gives about 2 oz. per person).

COOKING METHOD

1. Fit steamer basket in a medium saucepan. Add a cup or two of water; cover and bring to a boil.
2. Season the leaves with salt and pepper.
3. Steam for 5 to 7 minutes or until wilted, but still very green. Remove to a plate to drain.
4. Heat a large skillet and add olive oil. Add chopped garlic and toss for 1 minute. Add the steamed leaves and stir to heat through. Taste for seasoning and doneness. Serve immediately.

NUTRITIONAL ANALYSIS

Per serving: 33 calories, 1 g protein, 3 g carbohydrates, 2 g fat, 0 g saturated fat, 261 mg sodium, 32 mg calcium, 1 mg iron, 187 RE Vitamin A, 17 mg Vitamin C, 2 mg Vitamin E, 1 g fiber

AT A GLANCE
(FOR SKILLED COOKS IN A HURRY)

Wash, season, and steam greens 5 to 7 minutes. Drain. Heat skillet with oil. Sauté chopped garlic. Add to greens; toss and serve.

Spaghetti Squash

Until you've actually tried one, it's hard to believe that this commonly available squash can take the place of a fine-thread pasta—but it does. This is an extremely simple dish to get you started on its use. Imagine a pasta look-a-like with so few carbohydrates that tastes so good! This makes a good side dish or a vegetarian supper for two.

INGREDIENTS

1	SPAGHETTI SQUASH (3 c.)
2 cups	PREPARED LOW-SODIUM SPAGHETTI SAUCE
1 cup	SLICED MUSHROOMS
2 Tablespoons	CHOPPED PARSLEY
2 Tablespoons	PARMESAN CHEESE

COOKING METHOD

1. Preheat the oven to 400°F. Wash the outside of the squash and pierce it a few times with a fork. Set on a baking sheet and bake 1 hour or until very tender when tested with a fork. Cool.
2. Cut the cooked squash in half lengthwise and remove the seeds. Scrape the spaghetti-like threads out lightly with a fork and place in a baking dish. Toss with the low-sodium spaghetti sauce and mushrooms. Cover lightly with aluminum foil. Return to the oven for 20-30 minutes or until well heated through.
3. Scatter with parsley and Parmesan cheese and serve with a piece of bread and a salad for a hearty meal. It also makes a very tasty side dish with fish or chicken.

NUTRITIONAL ANALYSIS

Per serving: 125 calories, 4 g fat, 1 g saturated fat, 7% calories from saturated fat, 21 g carbohydrate, 4 g dietary fiber, 358 mg sodium.

AT A GLANCE
(FOR SKILLED COOKS IN A HURRY)

Preheat oven to 400°F. Wash outside of squash; pierce with a fork all over (5–6 times). Bake 1 hour (or 17 mins. microwave). Cool. Cut cooked squash in half lengthways and remove seeds. Lift/scrape squash threads out with a dinner fork, into bake dish. Toss with spaghetti sauce, mushrooms. Cover with foil. Return to oven 20–30 minutes. Garnish with parsley and cheese.

Pan Roasted Root Vegetables (Carrot, Rutabaga)

Throughout the fall and winter season, the root vegetables are at their best, and we really enjoy them. The pan-roasting method is one of our favorites and concentrates the flavors wonderfully. Root vegetables also keep well (for a week or more) out of refrigeration, which helps!

INGREDIENTS

1 pound	RUTABAGA
1 pound	CARROTS
Note: Also available are PARSNIPS, TURNIPS, WINTER SQUASH (several varieties)	
season	SALT
season	WHITE PEPPER
1 Tablespoon	NONAROMATIC OLIVE OIL
2 Tablespoons	PARSLEY, chopped

BEFORE YOU COOK:

Wash well, then peel (you can expect about 10–12 oz. of trim, so save it for stock—see p. 37, n. 5). Cut to get even sizes with some flat surfaces (keep sizes fairly large—2 in. x 1 in.).

COOKING METHOD

1. Heat a large skillet. Add oil to warm. Add vegetables and toss well. Spread out into a single layer and cover.
2. Adjust heat to medium-high and toss every 5 minutes or so. Watch so they don't over brown.
3. After 20 minutes, test for doneness with a sharp fork. Season with salt and pepper to taste. Add parsley and toss again before serving.

NUTRITIONAL ANALYSIS

Per serving: 120 calories, 3 g protein, 21 g carbohydrates, 4 g fat, .5 g saturated fat, 4% calories from saturated fats, 366 mg sodium, 87 mg calcium, 1 mg iron, 2,940 RE Vitamin A, 32 mg Vitamin C, 2 mg Vitamin E, 6 g fiber

AT A GLANCE
(FOR SKILLED COOKS IN A HURRY)

Wash and peel (save trim for stock). Cut into even sizes with flat surfaces. Heat pan and oil; sauté covered for 20 minutes. Season to taste. Add parsley and serve.

Steamed Green Vegetables (Broccoli)

We've used our favorite green vegetable to describe the method to use for broccoli, Brussels sprouts, asparagus, and green beans. While the times vary by a minute or two, the method remains the same. Our steamer is a vital part of the kitchen (see Equipment, p. 40, n. 1).

INGREDIENTS

8 ounces	BROCCOLI (1 typical bunch)	
season	SALT	
season	WHITE PEPPER	
1/2 teaspoon	BASIL, dried	

BEFORE YOU COOK:

Wash well. Trim off the very end pieces. Cut away but keep the bottom four inches of stalks.

COOKING METHOD

1. Bring the steamer to a boil. Add the stalks only. Season lightly with salt, pepper, and a scattering of the herbs.
2. Cover and steam for 5 minutes.
3. Add the tops and season as above. Cover and steam 10 minutes until tender and still very green.

NUTRITIONAL ANALYSIS

Per serving: 16 calories, 2 g protein, 7 g carbohydrates, 0 g fat, 0 g saturated fat, 0% calories from saturated fats, 149 mg sodium, 41 mg calcium, 1 mg iron, 59 RE Vitamin A, 39 mg Vitamin C, 1 mg Vitamin E, 2 g fiber

AT A GLANCE
(FOR SKILLED COOKS IN A HURRY)

Wash. Trim ends and last 4 inches of stalk. Season and steam stalks 5 minutes. Add tops and steam another 10 minutes.

Spinach Defrosted in Broth

This defrosting method is great for other frozen vegetables as well.

INGREDIENTS

1 cup	LOW-SODIUM CHICKEN OR VEGETABLE BROTH
1 10-oz. package	FROZEN SPINACH (1 1/2 c.)
1/8 teaspoon	GROUND NUTMEG
2 teaspoons	CORNSTARCH mixed with 2 Tablespoons water (slurry)

COOKING METHOD

1. Bring the broth to a boil in a small saucepan. Add the spinach, cover, reduce the heat to low, and cook for 10 minutes.
2. Add nutmeg. Pour in the slurry to thicken and heat for 30 seconds. Serve with a colorful vegetable such as carrots or tomatoes.

NUTRITIONAL ANALYSIS

Per serving: 34 calories, 0 g fat, 0% calories from fat, 0 g saturated fat, 0% calories from saturated fat, 6 g carbohydrates, 97 mg sodium, 2 g dietary fiber

Potato Diamonds-in-the-Jacket

SERVES 2 (EASILY MULTIPLIED)

Here is one of our most-often-served potato dishes. It is simple, yet delicious and unusual. Its portion size covers the plate but with less starch than normal. An all-the-way-round winner! P.S. You will need a microwave oven.

INGREDIENTS

1 8-ounce	IDAHO RUSSET BAKING POTATO
1 teaspoon	NONAROMATIC OLIVE OIL
1 teaspoon	I CAN'T BELIEVE IT'S NOT BUTTER® (light)
1 teaspoon	CHOPPED PARSLEY
season	SALT, PEPPER, PAPRIKA

BEFORE YOU COOK:

Wash the potato. Finely chop the parsley. Measure remaining ingredients.

COOKING METHOD

1. Microwave the potato for 6 minutes on high. Turn and cook 1 minute more.
2. Cut the potato in half lengthways and cut down into the inner flesh, making a one-inch deep diamond pattern. Squeeze gently to open the cuts.
3. Season lightly with salt, pepper, and paprika. Brush the surface with olive oil and set the cut side down in a frying pan over medium-high heat to brown (about 3 to 4 mins.).
4. Squeeze again to open cuts; brush with butter substitute. Dust with parsley and serve.

NUTRITIONAL ANALYSIS

Per serving: 152 calories, 3 g protein, 29 g carbohydrates, 3 g fat, 1 g saturated fat, 6% calories from saturated fats, 326 mg sodium, 14 mg calcium, 2 mg iron, 20 RE Vitamin A, 16 mg Vitamin C, 1 mg Vitamin E, 3 g fiber

Mashed Sweet Potatoes

SERVES 4

Sweet potatoes are clearly high in natural sugars; however, they are also chuck full of other nutrients, especially vitamin A, so we need to make room for them. Use this recipe as a vegetable side dish for a very low carbohydrate balance to a meal—a nice piece of fish or poultry and good greens with a broiled tomato. Boy, won't that look pretty!

INGREDIENTS

4 small to medium	ORANGE-COLORED SWEET POTATOES to make 2 cups
2 teaspoons	FRESH THYME LEAVES or 3/4 teaspoon dried thyme
1/4 teaspoon	SALT
1/4 teaspoon	PEPPER

COOKING METHOD
Peel and cut the sweet potatoes into 1/2-inch slices. Cook in a steamer over boiling water until tender, about 20 minutes. When they are very soft, tip into a bowl and mash with a fork or potato masher. Stir in thyme, salt, and pepper and serve.

NUTRITIONAL ANALYSIS
Per serving: 155 calories, 0 g fat, 0 g saturated fat, 0% calories from saturated fat, 37 g carbohydrates, 5 g fiber, 155 mg sodium.

Italian Bread with Roasted Vegetables

SERVES 12
SERVING: 1 WEDGE

I've mentioned this bread as a side dish for a simple "small" supper. It is so delicious it should come with a warning notice to limit the portion size! One wedge (1/12 of a 10.5-inch diameter round) is 24 grams of carbohydrate, so enjoy but be cautious! I make it in a 10.5-inch x 2-inch deep skillet, but you can choose your own loaf pan.

1 cup	WATER	2–2 3/4 cups	ALL-PURPOSE FLOUR
1 teaspoon	DRY YEAST	1	SWEET ONION, 1-inch pieces
1 teaspoon	OLIVE OIL	1	RED BELL PEPPER, 1-inch pieces
1/2 teaspoon	DRIED OREGANO	2 cloves	GARLIC, peel on
1/2 teaspoon	DRIED BASIL	6	SUNDRIED TOMATO halves, in strips
1/2 teaspoon	SALT	1/16 teaspoon	SEA SALT, kosher or ground

BEFORE YOU COOK:

Peel and chop the onion and pepper, and peel and crush the garlic. Cut the sundried tomatoes in fine strips. Measure the remaining ingredients.

METHOD OF ASSEMBLY

1. Sprinkle the yeast over the warm water in a large bowl and let set until creamy, about 10 minutes. Stir in the oregano, basil, and salt. Add 2 cups of the flour and mix thoroughly, adding more flour until you have a nice medium-firm dough. Turn out onto a floured surface and knead until the dough is smooth and springy, at least 5 minutes. Place the dough in an oiled bowl, cover, and allow to rise until doubled in volume, about 1 1/2 to 2 hours.
2. Preheat the oven to 425°F. Toss onions, peppers, and unpeeled garlic with 1/2 teaspoon of oil in a baking dish. Sprinkle with 1/8 teaspoon of salt. Bake 25 minutes or until the vegetables are tender and the garlic is soft. Cool before using. Peel the garlic and cut into small pieces.
3. Preheat the oven to 400°F. Spread the dough into a large rectangle. Scatter the vegetable mixture evenly over the top. Add the sun-dried tomato pieces and fold in the sides. Knead the vegetables into the dough until they are well distributed throughout. Pat the dough into a greased 10.5-inch skillet or pie pan. Allow it to rise about 30 minutes.
4. Make deep dimples in the dough with your fingertips. Drizzle the remaining 1/2 teaspoon oil over the top and sprinkle with the kosher salt. Bake 30 minutes or until golden brown. Cool on a rack before cutting.

NUTRITIONAL ANALYSIS

Per wedge: 116 calories, 3 g protein, 24 g carbohydrate, 1 g fat, 0 g saturated fat, 0% calories from saturated fat, 91 mg sodium, 2 g dietary fiber

AT A GLANCE:
(FOR SKILLED COOKS IN A HURRY)

Warm yeast in large bowl 10 minutes, add herbs and salt. Add flour, mix well to firm dough, knead 5 minutes. Pour in an oiled covered bowl until doubled (1 1/2 - 2 hrs.). Roast vegetables at 425°F 25 minutes, cool. Reduce oven to 400°F. Spread out dough, scatter on vegetables, fold over to distribute evenly, mould for pan or skillet (grease pan). Dimple the top, add oil and sea salt. Bake 30 minutes, cool and cut.

Recipes

SEAFOOD

Tilapia Pan Fried in Breadcrumbs

SERVES 2

*Tilapia is a moderately sized freshwater fish native to Israel where it has been fished for at least twenty-five hundred years. It is firm, white fish with a fresh, clean, non-fishy aroma, and when filleted for supermarket sale . . . **without bones.** They are commercially farmed and reasonably priced . . . all of this should make them wildly popular!*

INGREDIENTS

2 x 4 ounces	TILAPIA FILLETS
2 Tablespoons	FLOUR
1/2 teaspoon	SALT
1/4 teaspoon	PEPPER
1/2 teaspoon	DILL WEED
1	EGG (or 4 Tbsp. Egg Beaters™)
5 Tablespoons	TOASTED PLAIN BREADCRUMBS
spray	OLIVE OIL SPRAY
1	LEMON

BEFORE YOU COOK:

Rinse fish and allow to come to room temperature. Measure flour, eggs, and breadcrumbs in three separate dishes (oblong plastic trays from the seafood department work well). Season the flour and beat the egg. Cut the lemon into wedges.

COOKING METHOD

1. Preheat a heavy-based skillet to medium high (300°F).
2. Using a pair of tongs, dip the fillets back and front in the seasoned flour.
3. Dip into the eggs to completely coat. Finally, flop the fillets into the breadcrumbs. Use a spoon to ensure complete coverage.
4. Spray the pan and both sides of the fish with olive oil.
5. Fry for 3 minutes, then turn for another 2 minutes. Internal temperature should reach 160°F. Serve immediately with lemon wedges.

NUTRITIONAL ANALYSIS WITH EGG

Per serving: 248 calories, 24 g protein, 18 g carbohydrates, 9 g fat, 1 g saturated fat, 511 mg sodium, 84 mg calcium, 4 mg iron, 84 RE Vitamin A, 4 mg Vitamin C, 2 mg Vitamin E, 1 g fiber

NUTRITIONAL ANALYSIS WITH EGG BEATERS

Per serving: 225 calories, 24 g protein, 18 g carbohydrates, 6 g fat, .5 g saturated fat, 529 mg sodium, 81 calcium, 3 iron, 54 RE Vitamin A, 4 mg Vitamin C, 1 mg Vitamin E, 1 g fiber

AT A GLANCE
(FOR SKILLED COOKS IN A HURRY)

Rinse fillets and dry—room temperature. Flour, egg, and crumb fillets. Shallow fry (medium high) 2 minutes; turn for another 3 minutes. Serve with lemon wedges.

Tilapia, Scallops, Shrimp Stir-Fry in Coconut Cream Sauce

*Now and again we have the need to celebrate: a birthday or anniversary—the occasions when we used to eat out! We now prefer to eat at home; in many cases our food is better and almost always the portions make more sense! This recipe is remarkable—quite a celebration for less than seven dollars a portion. Compare **that** to eating out!*

INGREDIENTS

4.5 ounces	TILAPIA FILLET
3 ounces	LARGE SCALLOPS, cut in half
3 ounces	RAW SHELLED SHRIMP, 41/50 size
4	WHITE MUSHROOMS (1-in. diameter)
2	GREEN ONIONS, fine sliced
1 Tablespoon	GINGERROOT, finely cut "toothpicks"
1	GARLIC CLOVE, crushed
8	BASIL, whole fresh leaves
1 Tablespoon	OLIVE OIL
1/2 cup	NONFAT HALF AND HALF CREAM
1/2 teaspoon	COCONUT EXTRACT (see Buying, p. 33, n. 26)
1/2 teaspoon	TABASCO SAUCE
1 teaspoon	ARROWROOT or cornstarch
1 cup	BABY SPINACH LEAVES, fresh and tightly packed

BEFORE YOU COOK:

Rinse all seafood in cold water and dry with paper towels. Cut mushrooms into quarters, stem included. Fine slice green onion and ginger. Crush the garlic. Measure remaining ingredients. Cut tilapia into one-inch pieces.

COOKING METHOD

1. Heat a large skillet to 200°F on medium high.
2. Warm the oil and add the green onion, garlic, and ginger. Shallow fry for one minute, stirring all the time.
3. Add shrimp, scallops, and tilapia. Stir well to mix with the seasonings.
4. Add mushrooms and stir again. Stir-fry for 4 minutes.

5. Draw the pan off the heat. Add half and half and basil leaves. Stir to combine and bring to a boil. Add Tabasco and coconut extract and stir in arrowroot moistened with water (see p. 37, n. 7).

6. Add spinach leaves and cover to allow the leaves to wilt, about 1 minute. Stir to combine, and serve with rice or quinoa (see pp. 92–93).

NUTRITIONAL ANALYSIS

Per serving: 281 calories, 31 g protein, 12 g carbohydrates, 11 g fat, 1 g saturated fat, 389 mg sodium, 81 mg calcium, 3 mg iron, 127 RE Vitamin A, 10 mg Vitamin C, 2 mg Vitamin E, 2 g fiber

AT A GLANCE
(FOR SKILLED COOKS IN A HURRY)

Heat large skillet and add oil. Sauté onion, garlic, and ginger. Add tilapia, shrimp, and scallops–toss and stir. Add mushrooms (stir fry 4 mins.). Add half and half; boil and then add hot sauce and coconut extract. Thicken. Add spinach–wilt and stir in. Serve with rice or quinoa.

Baked Tilapia with Mushrooms and Spinach

SERVES 2

Another freshwater tilapia dish because of both price and quality. We were delighted with this very simple idea and how quickly it comes together.

INGREDIENTS

6	WHITE MUSHROOMS, 1 inch
2 teaspoons	LEMON JUICE
1/2 teaspoon	DILL WEED
1/2 teaspoon	SALT, divided in half
1/4 teaspoon	WHITE PEPPER
spray	OLIVE OIL SPRAY
2 cups	BABY SPINACH LEAVES, tightly packed
1/4 cup	GREEN ONION, finely chopped
2 x 4.5 ounces	TILAPIA FILLETS
1/4 teaspoon	HERBS OF PROVENCE
1/4 teaspoon	SALT
1/2 teaspoon	PAPRIKA

BEFORE YOU COOK:

Preheat oven and bake dish to 425°. Slice mushrooms 1/4-inch thick, including stalk. Wash Tilapia in cold water and dry on paper towels. Measure remaining ingredients.

COOKING METHOD

1. Clean mushrooms with a soft brush and spray lightly with olive oil. Season with 1/4 teaspoon of the salt, lemon juice, and dill. It helps to do this on a plate.
2. Spray spinach lightly with oil and season with remaining 1/4 teaspoon of the salt and the white pepper. Set aside.
3. Heat a skillet to 200°. Toss in the mushrooms and green onions, and fry for 2 minutes. Add sprayed, seasoned spinach and stir to just wilt the spinach. Remove to a plate to keep warm.
4. Spray the tilapia with oil and season with herbs and salt. Sear quickly in the hot skillet for 30 seconds on each side.
5. Transfer the mushroom-spinach mixture to a baking dish, making 2 mounds. Top each with a seared tilapia filet, dust with paprika, spray with oil, and bake for 8 minutes (160°F internal temperature).

NUTRITIONAL ANALYSIS

Per serving: 145 calories, 23 g protein, 4 g carbohydrates, 5 g fat, 0 g saturated fat, 684 mg sodium, 73 mg calcium, 4 mg iron, 202 RE Vitamin A, 13 mg Vitamin C, 0 mg Vitamin E, 3 g fiber

AT A GLANCE
(FOR SKILLED COOKS IN A HURRY)

Slice mushrooms and spray with oil. Season with salt, white pepper, lemon juice, and dill weed. Add onions and sauté 2 minutes. Add spinach to wilt, and turn out. Season fish with salt, herbs, and paprika; spray with oil. Sear in hot pan. Mound vegetables twice; drape with seared fish; bake 8 minutes at 425°F to 160°F internal.

Poached Tilapia in Oil and Vinegar Broth

SERVES 2

I must admit I'm not a great fan of the microwave oven for certain foods, but I do love it for defrosting quickly, for heating small drinks, for many vegetables, and especially for its ability to poach fish brilliantly. It's worth it just for this one culinary masterpiece.

INGREDIENTS

4 Tablespoons	TREENA'S OIL AND VINEGAR DRESSING (see p. 84)	season season	SALT WHITE PEPPER
1 teaspoon	HERBS OF PROVENCE	2 teaspoons	CAPERS
8 Tablespoons	FILTERED WATER	1/2 teaspoon	ARROWROOT or
to cover	WAXED KITCHEN PAPER		cornstarch
2 x 4.5 ounces	TILAPIA FILLETS	tiny pinch	POWDERED SAFFRON

BEFORE YOU COOK:

Rinse tilapia in cold water; dry on paper towels and season. Measure remaining ingredients.

COOKING METHOD

1. Heat a large ceramic or glass baking dish in the microwave for 2 minutes. Add the dressing with the water and stir in the herbs.
2. Warm the dressing, but don't boil. Add the seasoned tilapia and cover with waxed paper pressed down over the fish. It should cover the whole dish.
3. Microwave on high for 4 minutes only. It should reach 160°F to 170°F.
4. Remove the fish to a warm plate and cover.
5. Drain the cooking liquid into a small saucepan. Add capers and saffron and bring to a boil. Remove from the heat and thicken with arrowroot moistened with water (see p. 37, n. 7).
6. It will look like melted butter. It looks and tastes wonderful poured over the fish.

NUTRITIONAL ANALYSIS

Per serving: 197 calories, 21 g protein, 3 g carbohydrates, 11 g fat, 1 g saturated fat, 539 mg sodium, 38 mg calcium, 27 RE Vitamin A, 1 mg Vitamin C, 1 mg Vitamin E, 0 g fiber

AT A GLANCE
(FOR SKILLED COOKS IN A HURRY)

Warm oil and vinegar/water with herbs in microwave bake dish. Add seasoned tilapia. Cover with waxed paper. Microwave on high power 4 minutes. Drain cooking liquid. Add saffron and capers. Thicken and serve over fish.

Baked White Fish, Southern Italian

SERVES 4

I ate this dish in Sicily in a beachside restaurant on a lovely spring day with a fisherman out in the tiny bay singing operatic arias. It was so good (the fish) that for awhile I lost interest in my surroundings!

INGREDIENTS

1 teaspoon	NONAROMATIC OLIVE OIL
2 cups	CHOPPED ONION
1 (4-in.)	SPRING FRESH ROSEMARY or 1 teaspoon dried
3 cloves	GARLIC, bashed and chopped
2 ribs	CELERY, chopped
2 (14 1/2-oz.)	CANS DICED TOMATOES IN PUREE
1/2 cup	NONALCOHOLIC DRY WHITE WINE
1/4 cup	ROUGHLY CHOPPED GREEN OLIVES
2 Tablespoons	CAPERS
1/8 teaspoon	CRUSHED CHILIES
1/8 teaspoon	FRESHLY GROUND BLACK PEPPER
4 (6-oz.)	TILAPIA OR OTHER FIRM WHITE FISH FILLETS
1/2 teaspoon	EXTRA-VIRGIN OLIVE OIL
1 Tablespoon	ARROWROOT mixed with
2 Tablespoons	NONALCOHOLIC WHITE WINE (slurry)
1 Tablespoon	CHOPPED FRESH PARSLEY

BEFORE YOU COOK:

Chop the onion into 1/4-inch dice. Chop the garlic and the parsley. Measure the remaining ingredients.

COOKING METHOD

1. Preheat the oven to 375°F. Heat the oil in a high-sided skillet on medium high. Cook the onions with the sprig of rosemary for 1 minute. Add the garlic and celery and cook 2 minutes. Pour in the tomatoes and wine and simmer 4 minutes.
2. Stir in the olives, capers, chilies, and pepper. Bury the fish fillets in the sauce, cover, and bake for 8 minutes or until the fish flakes.
3. Divide the fish fillets among four hot plates Stir the olive oil and slurry into the remaining sauce and heat to thicken slightly. Spoon over the fish fillets, sprinkle with chopped parsley, and serve with a crusty Italian bread like Roasted Vegetable Bread (see p. 104).

NUTRITIONAL ANALYSIS

Per serving: 289 calories, 45 g protein, 18 g carbohydrate, 4 g fat, 1 g saturated fat, 3% calories from saturated fat, 3 g dietary fiber

AT A GLANCE
(FOR SKILLED COOKS IN A HURRY)

Preheat oven to 375°. Heat pan and add oil. Sauté onion. Add rosemary. Add garlic and celery and sauté. Add tomatoes and wine; simmer 4 minutes. Add olives, capers, chilies, and pepper. Bury fish in sauce. Bake 8 minutes to flake. Remove fish. Add oil and slurry to sauce. Thicken. Spoon over fish. Add parsley. Serve with good bread.

Halibut, Northwestern Style

SERVES 4

This dish was created in the FareStart Kitchens in Seattle, a truly inspiring enterprise that trains "homeless people" to re-enter the working community as chef-wanna-be's. I was part of their "team" for several years, and I am still a great fan. The dish is colorful and quite simple to fix. Roasting garlic reduces its pungency and gives great depth of flavor.

INGREDIENTS

Roasted Garlic Sauce

1 head	GARLIC
1/2 cup	NONFAT YOGURT CHEESE (p. 38, n. 10)
pinch	TINY PINCH SAFFRON
1 teaspoon	EXTRA-VIRGIN OLIVE OIL
1 Tablespoon	FRESHLY SQUEEZED LEMON JUICE

Halibut

1 teaspoon	EXTRA-VIRGIN OLIVE OIL
3 cups	FISH STOCK (p. 223)
1 Tablespoon	CHOPPED PARSLEY
1/4 teaspoon	SALT
1 Tablespoon	FRESHLY SQUEEZED LEMON JUICE
pinch	SAFFRON
4 (6-oz.)	HALIBUT FILLETS
4	ROMA TOMATOES
1 Tablespoon	ARROWROOT mixed with
2 Tablespoons	FISH STOCK OR WATER (slurry)
3 Tablespoons	CHOPPED PARSLEY

BEFORE YOU COOK:

Crush garlic cloves for cooking sauce. Make fish stock (see p. 223). Chop parsley. Squeeze lemon. Cut tomatoes in 1/4-inch dice. Measure remaining ingredients.

COOKING METHOD

Garlic Sauce

1. Cut the root end off the head of garlic and wrap in foil. Roast for an hour in the 350°F pre-heated oven or until very soft. Remove and cool before pressing out the cooked flesh. You

should have 2 Tablespoons. Combine with the yogurt cheese, saffron, olive oil, and lemon juice. Set aside.

Fish

1. Stir the olive oil and garlic together in a small saucepan on medium heat. Cook until it starts to sizzle, about 2 minutes, then add 2 cups of the fish stock and parsley. Turn to high and reduce the liquid by half at a vigorous reducing boil, about 5 minutes. Strain into a skillet large enough to hold the fish fillets. Add the other cup of stock, salt, lemon juice, and saffron. Bring to a boil. Set the fillets in the stock and reduce the heat to medium. Cover with a sheet of waxed paper, cut to fit the pan. Simmer 5 minutes then turn and cook 2 minutes longer. Remove to four hot soup plates.
2. Toss the tomatoes into the boiling liquid to just heat through, about 1 minute. Stir in the slurry and parsley. It should thicken almost immediately. Spoon over the fish fillets and serve with a dollop of the garlic sauce. Scatter more chopped parsley over it if you like.

NUTRITIONAL ANALYSIS

Per serving: 301 calories, 42 g protein, 17 g carbohydrate, 7 g fat, 1 g saturated fat, 3% calories from saturated fat, 361 mg sodium, 241 mg calcium, 3 mg iron, 180 RE Vitamin A, 35 mg Vitamin C, and 2 mg Vitamin E, 2 g dietary fiber

AT A GLANCE
(FOR SKILLED COOKS IN A HURRY)

Roast garlic head at 350°F wrapped in foil for one hour. Cool. Squeeze out 2 Tablespoons puree. Mix with yogurt, saffron, oil, and lemon. Stir oil and garlic over medium heat. Add fish stock and parsley. Reduce 50 percent. Add to skillet. Add extra stock, saffron, lemon juice, and salt. Boil. Put fillets into stock. Reduce heat. Cover with waxed paper. Simmer 5 minutes. Turn for 2 more minutes. Remove (keep warm). Add tomatoes. Boil. Stir in slurry and parsley. Spoon over fish. Top with garlic "sauce."

Halibut with Mango Chutney

This dish works well with good fresh halibut or any other firm white fish fillet such as tilapia (cut time to 3 mins. each side). It can be cooked under a radiant grill or in a skillet. The mango chutney is a real treat and can help win over the reluctant seafood eater!

INGREDIENTS

Mango Chutney

1 (1 c.)	FRESH MANGO
2 (1/2 c.)	GREEN ONIONS
1 Tablespoon	PEELED, GRATED FRESH GINGERROOT
1/2 cup	FRUITY WHITE WINE (I prefer nonalcoholic blanc.)
1/4 teaspoon	CAYENNE PEPPER

Halibut

1/4 teaspoon	SALT
1/4 teaspoon	FRESHLY GROUND BLACK PEPPER
4 (6-oz.)	HALIBUT FILLETS
6 cups	ARUGULA LEAVES, washed and spun dry
2 Tablespoons	CHOPPED PARSLEY

BEFORE YOU COOK:

Peel the mango, then pit and finely dice. Chop the white part of the green onion finely. Grate the gingerroot. Measure the remaining ingredients.

COOKING METHOD

1. Combine the mango, onion, ginger, wine, and cayenne in a small saucepan. Bring to a boil over medium heat, then reduce the heat and simmer for 10 minutes. Remove from heat and set aside until ready to serve. You can make this ahead if you like.
2. Preheat the broiler (or skillet). Season the fish with the salt and pepper, then spray lightly with cooking oil spray. Place the fish on a broiler pan (or skillet) and spray lightly with cooking spray.
3. Broil or shallow fry the fillets for 4 minutes on each side, or until the flesh is no longer translucent and flakes easily.
4. Divide the arugula among six plates and lay a fish fillet on top of each. Heap a spoonful of mango chutney on the fish and sprinkle a little chopped parsley over all.

NUTRITIONAL ANALYSIS

Per serving: 227 calories, 37 g protein, 9 g carbohydrate, 4 g fat, 1 g saturated fat, 4% calories from saturated fat, 245 mg sodium, 143 mg calcium, 2 mg iron, 324 RE Vitamin A, 20 mg Vitamin C, and 2 mg Vitamin E, 2 g dietary fiber

AT A GLANCE
(FOR SKILLED COOKS IN A HURRY)

Boil mango, onion, ginger, wine, and cayenne in a small pan; reduce and simmer 10 minutes. Preheat pan/broiler. Season and oil fish, then broil or sauté 4 minutes each side until it flakes (just!). Divide salad. Lay fish on greens. Heap mango on top and dust with parsley. Serve.

Kedgeree Smoked Fish and Rice

SERVES 4

We developed this "leaner look" at the very rich Indian/Scottish dish in Aberdeen, Scotland, where we tested it on a local. His comment was (in a rich brogue), "Well ye can see that you're ney a stingy mon." Stingy is the description of a mean person—exemplified by one who doesn't add enough butter to a kedgeree. I didn't add any, but he didn't pick up on it! If you like smoked seafood and rice, you'll love this dish.

INGREDIENTS

1 cup	LONG-GRAIN WHITE RICE
pinch	SAFFRON
2 cups	1% MILK
1/2 cup	NONALCOHOLIC WHITE WINE
1/8 teaspoon	WHITE PEPPER
1	BAY LEAF
1 pound	FINNAN HADDIE (smoked haddock or halibut or other local smoked white fish)
1 Tablespoon	BUTTER-FLAVORED MARGARINE (soft tub)
1 Tablespoon	DRY MUSTARD POWDER
2 teaspoons	ARROWROOT mixed with
1 Tablespoon	WATER (slurry)
2 Tablespoons	CHOPPED FRESH CHIVES
2	HARD COOKED EGG WHITES, sliced (discard yolks)
1/8 teaspoon	GROUND RED PEPPER

BEFORE YOU COOK:

Hard boil (10 mins.—see p. 51) the eggs. Presoak the smoked fish in cold 2% milk for 30 minutes to reduce sodium.

COOKING METHOD

1. Cook rice according to package directions with the saffron.
2. Combine milk, wine, white pepper, and bay leaf in a high-sided skillet, and simmer 10 minutes. Lay pieces of Finnan Haddie in milk mixture, cover with waxed paper, and simmer 8 minutes. Remove fish to a plate. Strain and reserve the milk.
3. Flake the fish, removing bones and bits of connective tissue. Stir margarine and mustard into the milk, and reheat in the skillet. Add fish and rice, and simmer 5 minutes. Stir in the slurry. Add egg whites, chives, and red pepper.

NUTRITIONAL ANALYSIS

Per serving: 388 calories, 46 g carbohydrates, 4 g fat, 1 g saturated fat, 2% calories from saturated fat, 721 mg sodium, 1 g dietary fiber

*Note: The fats are extremely low, but the carbs could be a problem for you. If so, reduce the
rice by half. I like to add snow peas or water chestnuts to replace the volume loss of rice.*

AT A GLANCE
(FOR SKILLED COOKS IN A HURRY)

Boil rice with saffron. Combine milk, wine, seasoning (pepper only), and bay leaf. Cover.
Simmer 10 minutes. Add smoked fish. Cover with waxed paper. Simmer 8 minutes.
Remove fish, and strain cooking liquids. Flake the fish (discard skin and bones). Add
margarine and mustard to milk. Add fish and rice, and simmer 5 minutes. Add slurry. Stir
to "glisten." Add egg white slices, chives, and red pepper.

Poached Salmon— Hot and Cold

*I'm often asked to look back over my sixty (is it **really** that long?!) years in food and select the one dish that gave me the most pleasure. After several stabs at it, I've finally made a choice: A centre cut fillet of Scottish (Atlantic) salmon poached in a well-seasoned broth that the French call court-bouillon then cooled, usually in the same liquid, and served over fresh salad greens in a lighter-styled mayonnaise. On the side, some very small new potatoes (or fingerlings). Pure bliss! So here it is again–just for you! Served best out of pan or cold, it's perfection!*

INGREDIENTS

1 pound	CENTRE CUT FRESH SALMON
1 teaspoon	OLIVE OIL
1 Tablespoon	GINGERROOT
1 bunch	GREEN ONIONS
2 Tablespoons	LEMON JUICE
1 teaspoon	DILL WEED
1 teaspoon	SEA SALT
2 Tablespoons	UNSALTED BUTTER, melted
2 teaspoons	SMALL CAPERS
2 Tablespoons	GOOD "LIGHT" MAYONNAISE (if serving cold)

BEFORE YOU COOK:

Rinse salmon briefly. Dry on paper towels. Finely chop or grate the ginger. Chop the green onion. Measure remaining ingredients.

COOKING METHOD

1. In a sauté pan, heat oil and toss together the ginger and green onions for 2 minutes. Add the lemon juice, dill, and salt with enough cold, *filtered* water to just cover the salmon (about 2 c.) in a microwave-safe glass or china dish.
2. Add the salmon and cover with the seasoned liquid. Place a sheet of waxed paper onto the surface.
3. Microwave on high for 5 minutes only. Remove salmon and cut in four pieces to serve hot with a *little* melted butter and capers. If you want to serve it cold, place in the fridge to cool rapidly in the liquid. Drain. Quarter. Serve with mayonnaise.

NUTRITIONAL ANALYSIS

Per serving hot with butter: 201 calories, 23 g protein, 0 g carbohydrates, 12 g fat, 5 g saturated fat, 277 mg sodium, 48 mg calcium, 1 mg iron, 73 RE Vitamin A, 1 mg Vitamin C, 0 g fiber

Per serving cold with light mayonnaise: 172 calories, 23 g protein, 1 g carbohydrates, 9 g fat, 2 g saturated fat, 333 mg sodium, 46 mg calcium, 1 mg iron, 16 RE Vitamin A, 1 mg Vitamin C, 2 mg Vitamin E, 0 g fiber

AT A GLANCE
(FOR SKILLED COOKS IN A HURRY)

Prepare *court bouillon.* Sauté ginger and onions in oil. Add lemon, dill, and filtered water. Place rinsed salmon into microwave dish. Add 2 cups liquid. Cover with waxed paper. Microwave on high for 5 minutes. Serve hot with a little butter and capers, or cool in bouillon and serve with a light mayonnaise.

Baked Salmon in a Jacket

SERVES 2

*This is a fun and fast supper dish, providing you have a microwave to bake the potato swiftly. We began this idea as a treat after a long drive in our motor home. We used canned sockeye salmon (with lower sodium content), but you can just as easily use any canned meat, poultry, or beans for a vegetarian protein. Try 4 ounces of tofu with shitake mushrooms if you **really** want to experiment! The baked potato half will generally be an acceptable carbohydrate serving. A good salad on the side makes an attractive whole meal.*

INGREDIENTS

1 large	"IDAHO" RUSSET BAKING POTATO
1 8-ounce can	SOCKEYE SALMON (lower sodium)
1/2 teaspoon	WHITE PEPPER
1 Tablespoon	CHOPPED FRESH CHIVES
spray	OLIVE OIL SPRAY
dust	PAPRIKA

BEFORE YOU COOK:

Wash the baking potato. Open the can and drain off the juices. Chop the chives. Measure remaining ingredients.

COOKING METHOD

1. Microwave the potato for 6 minutes on high. Turn over and give it one minute more. Allow to cool.
2. Cut the potato in half lengthways and carefully scoop out the cooked center.
3. Mix the canned salmon with the potato, pepper, and chives, and pile back until it heaps into the empty potato skin.
4. Spray with olive oil and dust with paprika. Bake at 350° for 10 minutes to "gracefully" reheat, or zap it for another 2 minutes on high in the microwave (if you must!).

NUTRITIONAL ANALYSIS

Per serving: 341 calories, 22 g protein, 29 g carbohydrates, 12 g fat, 3 g saturated fat, 79 mg sodium, 271 mg calcium, 3 mg iron, 41 RE Vitamin A, 16 mg Vitamin C, 3 mg Vitamin E, 3 g fiber

Shrimp 'n' Greens

The greens in this swift recipe can be your choice of collards, kale, turnip tops, mustard, but not the fine-textured spinach or Swiss chard, which lose much of their volume in cooking. When all the ingredients are as fresh as possible, this dish is a real celebration.

INGREDIENTS

10 ounces	LEAFY GREENS	1/4 teaspoon	CAYENNE PEPPER
1 cup	CHICKEN STOCK	2 cloves	GARLIC
2 tsps. divided	HERBS OF PROVENCE	1/2 pound	SHRIMP, shell off
spray	OLIVE OIL SPRAY	2 teaspoons	THAI FISH SAUCE (optional)
1/4 pound	MUSHROOMS	2 teaspoons	ARROWROOT or cornstarch
1 teaspoon	LEMON JUICE		

BEFORE YOU COOK:

Wash greens and slice into 1/2-inch x 2-inch pieces. Slice mushrooms in fat pieces (1/2-in.). Crush garlic. Rinse shrimp and dry on paper towels. Measure remaining ingredients.

COOKING METHOD

1. Simmer the greens in chicken stock with 1 teaspoon of the Herbs of Provence in a covered saucepan for 15 minutes or until tender. Drain well and retain the cooking liquid.
2. Heat skillet, spray with oil, and sauté mushrooms with lemon juice and cayenne about 2 minutes. Turn out onto a plate.
3. Reheat skillet, spray with oil, and sauté garlic briefly. Add shrimp with the remaining 1 teaspoon of Herbs of Provence. Toss for 3 minutes. Add fish sauce if you are using it, mushrooms, and greens. Stir to heat. Add enough of the greens cooking liquid to moisten, then thicken with arrowroot (see p. 37, n. 7).

Note: If you use fish sauce, you will not need to add salt.

NUTRITIONAL ANALYSIS

Per serving: 215 calories, 30 g protein, 9 g carbohydrates, 4 g fat, 1 g saturated fat, 696 mg sodium, 202 mg calcium, 4 mg iron, 783 RE Vitamin A, 28 mg Vitamin C, 2 mg Vitamin E, 4 g fiber

AT A GLANCE
(FOR SKILLED COOKS IN A HURRY)

Simmer greens with herbs in chicken stock for 15 minutes. Reserve liquid. Sauté mushrooms with lemon and cayenne. Turn out. Sauté shrimp with garlic and herbs. Combine greens, mushrooms, shrimp, optional fish sauce. Moisten with greens' liquid. Thicken and serve.

Shrimp Gumbo

Gumbo just happened—the ingredients grew in abundance and the shrimp were there for the taking. The smokey bacon, garlic, and okra got on so well with the hot peppers and the oil or lard—the only problem was their need for energy came from the fat and sometimes robust portions. With careful trimming, this is still great eating.

INGREDIENTS

1 pound	MEDIUM SHRIMP (uncooked, in the shell)
1 cup	UNCOOKED LONG GRAIN WHITE RICE
3 teaspoons	NONAROMATIC OLIVE OIL, divided
1/4 pound	CANADIAN BACON
1 1/2 cups	CHOPPED ONION
2 cloves	GARLIC, bashed and chopped
1 cup	CELERY
1	LARGE RED BELL PEPPER, cut in 1/4-inch dices (generous cup)
3 Tablespoons	TOMATO PASTE
1/4 cup	ALL-PURPOSE FLOUR
2 cups	FROZEN OR FRESH SLICED OKRA (1/2-in. slices)
4 cups, divided	SHRIMP-SHELL STOCK
1/4 teaspoon	CAYENNE PEPPER
1/2 teaspoon	DRIED THYME
2	BAY LEAVES
1 teaspoon	GUMBO FILÉ

BEFORE YOU COOK:

Peel the shrimp but keep the shells and boil them in 4 cups water for 2 minutes. Strain and discard shells. Use 2 cups shrimp stock to cook the rice—boil, reduce heat, simmer with lid on for 15 minutes. Cut Canadian bacon into 1/2-inch dice, chop onion, crush garlic, cut celery into 1/2-inch dice, and cut red pepper in 1/4-inch dice. Measure remaining ingredients.

COOKING METHOD

1. Heat 1 teaspoon of the oil in a skillet or chef's pan on medium high. Sauté the Canadian bacon 2 minutes. Add the onions and cook 2 minutes. Add the garlic, celery, and red pepper and continue to sauté 3 to 4 minutes. Pull the vegetables to the side of the pan and add the tomato paste. Cook, stirring, until it darkens, then stir to coat the vegetables. Remove to a plate.

2. Heat the remaining oil in the same pan. Shake the okra in the flour in a bag. Sieve off any extra flour. Brown the floured okra in the hot oil. Return the vegetables to the pan and add the remaining 2 cups of shrimp-shell stock. Season with the cayenne, thyme, and bay leaves, and simmer until the okra is tender, about 10 minutes. Stir in the shrimp. Add the filé and simmer 2 minutes until thickened.

3. Divide the rice among four hot soup plates and pour the gumbo over the top. Garnish with chopped fresh parsley if you like.

NUTRITIONAL ANALYSIS

Per serving: 419 calories, 60 g carbohydrate, 7 g fat, 2 g saturated fat, 4% calories from saturated fat, 570 mg sodium, 6 g fiber

AT A GLANCE
(FOR SKILLED COOKS IN A HURRY)

(Follow "before you cook" for shrimp-shell stock and rice.)

Heat oil; brown bacon 2 minutes. Add onion—then garlic, celery, and red pepper; sauté 3 to 4 minutes. Pull vegetables to side of pan and brown tomato paste—6 to 7 minutes. Mix into vegetables and remove to plate. Add oil and brown floured okra. Return vegetables and add shrimp stock. Season with cayenne, thyme, and bay. Simmer 10 minutes until okra tender. Add shrimp; stir in filé and simmer for 5 minutes. Serve over the rice.

Shrimp and Mushroom Risotto

There is a restaurant in Washington, D.C., that deserves to be the power-lunch or dinner center. The food is magnificent, and everything is organic. Now I'm neither a vegetarian nor an organic-only person, but I respect both as the ultimate swing of the pendulum. What I love about "Nora's" is that she has done the right thing in the right way. I got this recipe from Nora—thanks!

INGREDIENTS

Rice

1 teaspoon	NONAROMATIC OLIVE OIL
1/4 cup	FINE-CHOPPED SWEET ONION
5 large cloves	GARLIC, bashed and chopped
1 1/2 cups	ARBORIO RICE
2 cups	NONALCOHOLIC DRY WHITE WINE, divided
3 cups	LOW-SODIUM CHICKEN STOCK, divided
1/4 teaspoon	SAFFRON THREADS

Main Ingredients

4 teaspoons	NONAROMATIC OLIVE OIL, divided
3 cloves	GARLIC, bashed and chopped
1/2 pound	CREMINI MUSHROOMS
1 teaspoon	WILD MUSHROOM POWDER (optional)
2 Tablespoons	FRESHLY SQUEEZED LEMON JUICE, divided
1/2 teaspoon	SALT
1/4 teaspoon	PEPPER
1 pound	MEDIUM RAW SHRIMP
1 cup	LOW-SODIUM CHICKEN STOCK
1 cup	NONALCOHOLIC DRY WHITE WINE
1/2 bunch	SPINACH
1 cup	FROZEN PETIT PEAS
2 Tablespoons	CHOPPED CHIVES OR PARSLEY (for garnish)
6 Tablespoons	FRESH GRATED PARMESAN CHEESE (optional, adds 2 g. of fat per serving)

BEFORE YOU COOK:

Fine-chop the onion. Crush the garlic. Slice the mushrooms. Make wild mushroom powder (see p. 31, n. 13). Shell the raw shrimp. Cut washed stemmed spinach in thin strips and cut across to 2-inch length.

COOKING METHOD

1. Heat the oil in a skillet or chef's pan on medium high. Shallow fry the onion until tender and transparent, about 3 minutes. Add the garlic and cook 1 minute more. Stir in the rice and cook until it starts to look translucent, about 2 minutes. Combine the wine and stock in a saucepan and heat. Add 1 cup of the liquid to the rice and bring to a boil. Reduce the heat, add the saffron, and simmer until the liquid is absorbed. Keep adding liquid 1 cup at a time stirring frequently until the rice is al dente, about 20 minutes. Spread the rice on a baking sheet and cool.

2. Heat 3 teaspoons of the oil in the pan on medium high. Add the garlic and sauté 30 seconds, then toss in the mushrooms. Sprinkle with the mushroom powder and shallow fry until tender, 2 minutes. Season with the lemon juice, salt, and pepper. Tip out onto a plate.

3. Heat the remaining oil. Sauté the shrimp 2 minutes or until pink. Pour in the stock and wine. Return the mushrooms and rice to the pan to heat through. Stir in the peas and spinach and cook 2 minutes or until bright green. Sprinkle with the remaining lemon juice. Divide among six hot soup plates. Garnish with chives or parsley.

NUTRITIONAL ANALYSIS

Per serving: 321 calories, 48 g carbohydrate, 5 g fat, 1 g saturated fat, 3% calories from saturated fat, 411 mg sodium, 4 g dietary fiber. To reduce carbohydrates, halve the quantity of rice.

AT A GLANCE
(FOR SKILLED COOKS IN A HURRY)

Heat oil, sauté onion. Add garlic. Stir in rice and cook 2 minutes. Combine wine and stock in a pan and heat. Add 1 cup to rice—boil—and reduce. Add saffron. Simmer and stir. Add extra liquid until rice is cooked (20 mins.). Spread rice out to cool rapidly. Add oil to hot pan. Add garlic, mushrooms, and *optional* mushroom powder. Sauté. Season with lemon, salt, and pepper and turn out. Add more oil and heat. Sauté shrimp until pink (2 mins.). Add remaining stock/wine and return rice and vegetables. Add peas and spinach for 2 minutes. Serve with grated cheese (optional).

Pacific Paella

The Paella rightfully belongs to the Spanish people. All the classic local ingredients meet together to make this regional dish one of the world's best combination rice dishes. If you shift the method over to the Pacific Ocean, the local ingredients change and another great regional dish is possible. In a way, it's fusion, but this time with method and ingredients. By the way, I think it really works well.

INGREDIENTS

2	CHICKEN THIGHS
1 1/2 teaspoon	RESERVED CHICKEN FAT
1/2 pound	TUNA
1/2 pound	MEDIUM SHRIMP, peeled
1	ONION
1 clove	GARLIC
1	JALAPENO PEPPER
1 1/2 cups	FROZEN OR CANNED CORN NIBLETS
1	RED BELL PEPPER
1 cup	MEDIUM-GRAIN RICE
1/2 teaspoon	SALT
1/8 teaspoon	PEPPER
1/8 teaspoon	SAFFRON THREADS
2 cups	CANNED OR HOMEMADE LOW-SODIUM CHICKEN STOCK (p. 225)
1 1/2 pounds	ROMA TOMATOES
1	RECIPE GRAHAM'S COCONUT CREAM (pp. 109–110)
6 Tablespoons	CHOPPED CILANTRO (optional)

BEFORE YOU COOK:

Wash chicken and dry on paper towels. Cut tuna into 1-inch cubes. Peel and de-vein shrimp. Finely dice onion. Crush garlic. Seed and chop jalapeno. Seed and cut pepper into 1-inch dice. Peel and cut tomatoes into 1-inch pieces. Make Coconut Cream. Chop cilantro.

COOKING METHOD

1. Heat a chef's pan or high-sided skillet on medium high. Drop the chicken in, skin side down, and cook 7 minutes, turning several times to cook through. Remove to a plate and cover. Drain off the accumulated fat and put 1 teaspoon back into the hot pan. Cook the tuna and shrimp 2 minutes. Tip onto the plate with the chicken.

2. Pour 1/2 teaspoon of the accumulated chicken fat into the hot pan still on medium high. Sauté the onion, garlic, and jalapeno pepper, 3 minutes or until the onion wilts. Add the corn and cook, stirring to carmelize the corn, 2 minutes. Stir in the bell pepper and rice. Season with 1/2 teaspoon salt, 1/8 teaspoon pepper, and 1/8 teaspoon saffron. Pour in the stock, bring to a boil, cover, and reduce the heat to medium. Cook 20 minutes, shaking once or twice.

3. Remove and discard the skin and bones from the chicken and add the meat, fish, and tomatoes to the rice. Stir in the coconut cream. Heat through and serve from the pan or tip into a 3-quart bowl and pat down. Top with a large serving platter and turn upside down to mold into shape. This is quite a feat! Scatter the cilantro over the rice and serve in wedges.

NUTRITIONAL ANALYSIS

Per serving: 346 calories, 47 g carbohydrate, 8 g fat, 3 g saturated fat, 8% calories from saturated fat, 347 mg sodium, 4 g dietary fiber

AT A GLANCE
(FOR SKILLED COOKS IN A HURRY)

Heat large chef's pan (10–11 in. diameter, 2 in. deep). Put in chicken, skin down. Turn often for 7 minutes. Remove and cover. Drain fat. Return 1 teaspoon. Sauté tuna and shrimp 2 minutes. Remove. Cover. 1/2 teaspoon fat. Sauté onion, garlic, and jalapeno. Add corn and cook to slight brown. Add bell pepper and rice. Season. Add saffron. Add stock. Boil. Cover. Reduce heat. Cook 20 minutes. Shake occasionally. Skin and bone chicken. Add meat, fish, and tomatoes to rice. Add coconut cream. Serve.

Ensenada Seafood Stew with Roasted Tomato Salsa

SERVES 6

I hope you'll appreciate the health-giving properties of this stew and find, as our vendor advised, that it relieves you from "feeling tired." I have added to this traditional stew a creamy finish that distinguished a fine soup I was served in our wine-cask restaurant. In essence, it may remind you of a creamy version of a paella. Serve this with a mound of Saffron Rice (p. 94) and a bit of Roasted Tomato Salsa (p. 228).

INGREDIENTS

Stew

8 ounces	SQUID "STEAKS" (free of cartilage and tentacles) (your choice)
12	SMALL CLAMS in the shell
12 ounces	LARGE PRAWNS
6 ounces	ORANGE ROUGHY FILLET (or tilapia)
2 teaspoons	LIGHT OLIVE OIL
1	LARGE SWEET ONION, roughly chopped
3 cloves	GARLIC, peeled, bashed, and chopped
3	CARROTS, peeled and cut on the diagonal into 1/4-inch slices (1 c.)
3	STALKS CELERY, cut on the diagonal into 1/2-inch slices (1 c.)
1	RED BELL PEPPER, cored and cut into 1-inch strips
1 cup	MUSHROOMS, quartered
1/2 cup	DRY WHITE WINE (I prefer de-alcoholized chardonnay.)
1/2 cup	LOW-SODIUM FISH OR VEGETABLE STOCK (pp. 222–23)
1/4 teaspoon	SALT
1/4 teaspoon	FRESHLY GROUND BLACK PEPPER

Sauce

1 cup	YOGURT CHEESE (p. 38, n. 10)
1/4 cup	ARROWROOT
1/2 cup	DRY WHITE WINE (I prefer de-alcoholized chardonnay.)
2 cups	LOW-SODIUM FISH OR VEGETABLE STOCK (pp. 222–23)
3 Tablespoons	ROASTED TOMATO SALSA (p. 228), or to taste

Garnish

1/4 cup	CILANTRO, chopped

Vegetarian Option

2 small	COOKED ARTICHOKE HEARTS, fresh or canned, cut in half
2	CANNED HEARTS OF PALM, cut diagonally into 3 pieces

BEFORE YOU COOK

Note: If you are challenged by the idea of squid, please go ahead and replace it with seafood of your choosing.

1. Cut the squid into 1-inch squares. Cover with water in a small saucepan and cook over low heat for 25 minutes. (If the squid has been tenderized—it will be full of tiny holes made by tenderizing needles—it will cook tender in about 5 mins.) Strain and place the chopped squid in a pile on a large plate.
2. Scrub the clams and place in a frying pan with 1/4 cup water. Cover and bring to a boil. Remove from the heat as soon as the clams open, 3 to 5 minutes. When cool enough to handle, remove the meat from the shells. Place the clams in a separate pile on the plate with the squid.
3. Peel the prawns, leaving on the last bit of shell and the tail. If they haven't been previously deveined, make a shallow cut down the back of each prawn and remove the gritty digestive tract. Place the prawns on the plate with the squid and clams.
4. Cut the orange roughy fillet into 1-inch squares. Add to the plate with the other fish, cover, and refrigerate until ready to cook.

METHOD OF ASSEMBLY

1. Warm 1 teaspoon of the oil in a large high-sided skillet over medium-high heat. Sauté the onion for 2 minutes to release its flavorful oils. Toss in the garlic and cook for 1 more minute. Add the carrots, celery, pepper, and mushrooms. Stir for a minute or two, then add the wine.
2. Boil, uncovered, over medium-high heat until the carrots are tender, 10 to 12 minutes. Add up to 1/2 cup of the fish or vegetable stock as the liquid evaporates. (*Vegetarian Option:* Use vegetable stock here. Set aside 1/6 of this mixture for each vegetarian serving before proceeding to the next step.)
3. Heat the remaining 1 teaspoon of oil in a large saucepan or small Dutch oven. Add the prawns and orange roughy, sprinkle with the salt and pepper, and cook for 30 seconds. Gently stir in the cooked vegetables, clams, and squid. Remove from the heat while you prepare the sauce.

To Prepare the Sauce:

1. Spoon the yogurt cheese into a 4-cup measuring glass.
2. Mix the arrowroot with the wine to make a slurry. Combine the stock and the slurry in a saucepan and stir over medium heat until thick and glossy. (Vegetarian Option: Use vegetable stock here. Set aside 1/4 cup of sauce at the end of this step.) Pour a little of the hot, thickened stock into the yogurt cheese and mix well to temper the yogurt. Add the rest of the stock to the yogurt cheese and whisk until no pure white remains.

3. Pour the sauce over the fish and vegetables. Add salsa to your taste and heat very gently, not allowing the stew to boil.

To Serve:

Place a scoop of saffron rice in the center of a warmed dinner plate and surround the rice with a ring of stew. Garnish with the chopped cilantro and pass the remaining salsa for those, like Treena, who like it hot.

NUTRITIONAL ANALYSIS

Per serving: 289 calories, 30 g carbohydrate, 4 g fat, 1 g saturated fat, 13% calories from saturated fat, 3 g dietary fiber

Vegetarian Option: Hearts of Artichoke and Palm

When almost ready to serve, heat the reserved vegetable mixture in a small saucepan. Add the artichoke hearts and hearts of palm and heat through. Pour the reserved yogurt cheese sauce over the heated vegetables and season with salsa to taste. Heat very gently, not allowing it to boil.

Vegetarian Option Nutritional Profile per serving: 287 calories, 4 g fat, 0 g saturated fat, 57 g carbohydrate, 5 g dietary fiber

AT A GLANCE
(FOR SKILLED COOKS IN A HURRY)

Cook squid (if chosen) in small saucepan of water and simmer 25 minutes (if tenderized, 5 mins.). Open clams in skillet with 1/2 cup water. Cover. Boil (3 mins.) to open. Cool. Remove "meat." Discard shells. Prepare shrimp and cut orange roughy into 1-inch squares. Heat oil. Sauté onion. Add garlic. Then add all vegetables. Sauté/toss. Add wine. Boil 10–12 minutes (carrot tender). Add fish (or vegetable) stock if needed. In separate pan, heat oil. Sauté fish and shrimp with seasonings for 30 seconds only. Stir all into vegetables. Cover and set aside off heat.

Sauce

Spoon yogurt cheese into 4-cup measure. Thicken the stock. Pour 1/4 cup into cheese to "temper" (see notes). Then pour the thinned, warmed yogurt into the main dish to "cream" it. Add salsa. Taste. Reheat but don't boil. Serve.

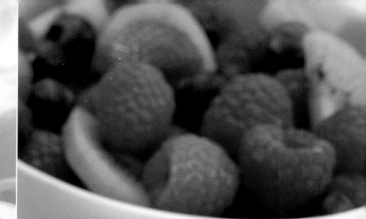

Whole Egg Omelet with Mushrooms and Bacon **pg. 54**

Pancakes — Extra Thin **pg. 57**

BREAKFAST AND BRUNCH **pg. 47**

Minestrone pg. 67

LUNCHES OR SUPPERS pg. 62

Spinach Salad with Pineapple and Avocado **pg. 69**

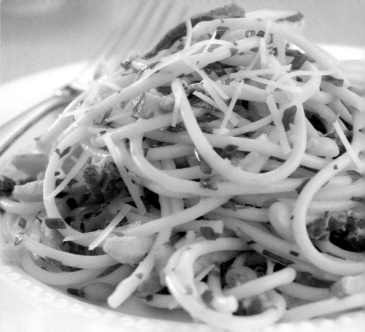

Spaghetti Carbonara **pg. 73**

Pasta with Mushrooms and Peas

pg. 75

Poached Salmon
Hot and Cold **pg. 122**

Roast Duck Breasts pg. 152

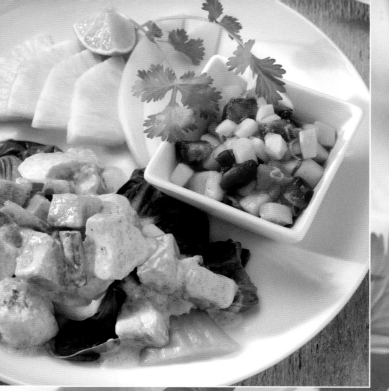

Curried Chicken with Sweet Potatoes and Bananas **pg. 173**

Thai Style Chicken **pg. 163**

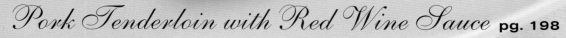

Pork Tenderloin with Red Wine Sauce **pg. 198**

MEATS pg. 175

Indian Ocean Gumbo

SERVES 4

Our visit to the Seychelles—an island group in the middle of the Indian Ocean—inspired this recipe. There's a remarkable mix of both Africa, India, and the French; what an amazing foundation for a great cuisine. I kept it simple, using shrimp (but all seafood can also be used). Cinnamon trees grow wild and vegetables flourish, as do coconuts and palm trees. No real need for okra!

INGREDIENTS

1/4 cup	ALL-PURPOSE FLOUR
1/8 teaspoon	GROUND CINNAMON
1 pound	SMALL SHRIMP (raw in shell) (51 to 60 shrimp per pound)
1 cup	LONG-GRAIN WHITE RICE
1/16 teaspoon	SAFFRON POWDER
1/2 teaspoon	SALT
2 teaspoons	NONAROMATIC OLIVE OIL
1	LARGE ONION
2 cloves	GARLIC
1	RED BELL PEPPER
1	GREEN BELL PEPPER
1/4 cup	TOMATO PASTE
1 teaspoon	DRIED THYME
1/2 teaspoon	CAYENNE PEPPER
2	TURKISH BAY LEAVES
4 cups	LOW-SODIUM CHICKEN STOCK (p. 225)
1 (15-oz.) can	PALM HEARTS, cut in 1-inch lengths
1/4 cup	COCONUT CREAM (optional)
2	SMALL GREEN ONIONS
1 Tablespoon	CHOPPED FRESH PARSLEY

BEFORE YOU COOK:

Peel shrimp. Keep "shells." Finely chop onion. Crush garlic. Cut both peppers into 1-inch squares. Chop green onions and parsley.

COOKING METHOD

1. Preheat the oven to 400°F. Combine the flour and cinnamon; place in a glass pie plate and bake 8 minutes. Set aside. Shell the shrimp, reserving the shells. Bring the shells to a boil

in a saucepan with 2 cups water and simmer 20 minutes. Strain, reserving the water in a saucepan; add the rice, saffron, and 1/4 teaspoon of the salt and bring to a boil. Reduce the heat to simmer and cook, uncovered, 15 minutes. Cover and keep warm.

2. Heat 1 teaspoon oil in a high-sided skillet on medium high. Sauté the onion 8 minutes or until golden brown. Add the garlic and roasted flour cinnamon and sauté 2 minutes more. Remove to a bowl and set aside.

3. Add the remaining 1 teaspoon oil to the pan and fry the peppers 1 minute. Add the tomato paste and continue cooking until it darkens, about 2 minutes. Stir in the onion flour mixture and add the thyme, cayenne, and bay. Continue cooking for 5 minutes, stirring so the flour won't burn. Pour the stock in slowly, stirring constantly to prevent any lumps from forming. When it comes to a boil, add the palm hearts, shrimp, and remaining salt, and simmer 3 minutes.

4. Place 1/2 cup rice in each of four preheated bowls. Spoon the gumbo over the rice and add a dollop of the coconut cream. Scatter the onions and parsley on top.

NUTRITIONAL ANALYSIS

Per serving: 405 calories, 27 g protein, 62 g carbohydrate, 6 g fat, 1 g saturated fat, 1% calories from saturated fat, 790 mg sodium, 6 g dietary fiber

AT A GLANCE
(FOR SKILLED COOKS IN A HURRY)

Preheat oven 400°F. Brown flour/cinnamon (8 mins.). Set aside. Shell shrimp. Cook shells in 2 cups water. Boil for 20 minutes. Strain, discard shells. Cook rice in shrimp stock (15 mins.) with salt and saffron. Heat oil in skillet. Sauté onion; add garlic and browned flour. Stir well. Remove to a bowl. Add oil. Sauté peppers. Add tomato paste. Cook to darken (see notes). Add seasonings. Stir well. Add stock slowly; stir out lumps. Bring to boil. Reduce heat. Add shrimp, palm hearts and salt. Garnish with coconut cream and parsley.

Recipes

POULTRY

Chicken Curry Sri Lankan Style

We visited Sri Lanka at a time of relative peace during their protracted time of civil unrest. It is a beautiful land with a heady aromatic cuisine—slightly sweet, warmly aromatic. We were given the recipe for their local curry mix and this recipe, which includes a red wine in the cooking liquid. The result is really unusual and pleasant.

INGREDIENTS

6	BONELESS, SKINLESS CHICKEN THIGHS
1 teaspoon	NONAROMATIC OLIVE OIL
1 large	ONION, roughly chopped
2 cloves	GARLIC, bashed and chopped
1 teaspoon	SRI LANKA CURRY (see recipe on the next page)
1 teaspoon	BROWN SUGAR
1/2 teaspoon	SALT
1	SERRANO CHILI, finely sliced with seeds
4	ROMA TOMATOES, chopped in 1/4-inch pieces
1 cup	LOW-SODIUM CHICKEN STOCK (p. 225)
1 cup	NONALCOHOLIC RED WINE
1 Tablespoon	CORNSTARCH mixed with 2 Tablespoons nonalcoholic red wine (slurry)
1/4 cup	YOGURT CHEESE (p. 38, n. 10)
2 Tablespoons	CHOPPED FRESH MINT
2 Tablespoons	CHOPPED FRESH CILANTRO
2 Tablespoons	CHOPPED FRESH PARSLEY
1 cup	COOKED LONG GRAIN BROWN RICE

BEFORE YOU COOK:

Trim off excess visible fat. Rinse the chicken and dry on paper towels. Chop the onion, bash and chop garlic, chop tomatoes in 1/4-inch pieces. Chop the fresh herbs.

COOKING METHOD

1. Heat a high-sided skillet and add oil. Fry the onion until it starts to wilt, about 2 minutes, then add the garlic, curry, brown sugar, salt, and chili. Reduce the heat and cook until the onions are soft, 12–15 minutes. Stir in the tomatoes. Lay the chicken pieces on top, pour in the stock and wine, cover, and simmer 45 minutes.

2. Push the chicken pieces aside and stir the slurry into the liquid. Let it boil for 30 seconds to cook the starch. Stir some of the hot liquid into the yogurt cheese to temper it, then pour it into the pan. Combine the fresh herbs and add half to the curry.
3. Serve on a bed of rice. Scatter the remaining spearmint, cilantro, and parsley over the whole plate.

Curry Mix

1 teaspoon	GROUND NUTMEG
1/2 teaspoon	GROUND CINNAMON
1/2 teaspoon	FRESHLY GROUND BLACK PEPPER
1/2 teaspoon	GROUND CARDAMOM
1/2 teaspoon	GROUND RED PEPPER
1/8 teaspoon	GROUND CLOVES
1/2 teaspoon	GROUND MUSTARD

Combine the spices in a small bowl for use in the dish. You may want to multiply the mix by 10 and use it elsewhere.

NUTRITIONAL ANALYSIS

Per serving: 357 calories, 38 protein, 26 g carbohydrate, 9 g fat, 2 g saturated fat, 5% calories from saturated fat, 485 mg sodium, 63 mg calcium, 3 mg iron, 148 RE Vitamin A, 45 mg Vitamin C, 1 mg Vitamin E, 4 g dietary fiber

AT A GLANCE
(FOR SKILLED COOKS IN A HURRY)

Heat oil and sauté onion. Add garlic, curry powder, brown sugar, salt, and chili. Reduce heat and cook onion tender (12–15 mins.). Stir in tomatoes, lay chicken on top, and add stock and wine. Cover, simmer 45 minutes. Set chicken aside. Thicken with slurry. Add small amount thickened liquid to temper the yogurt cheese; stir. Add to main pan with salt, half the herbs, and chicken. Heat but don't boil. Dust with herbs. Serve over rice.

Hawaiian Curried Chicken

Hawaii has an intriguing mix of cultures. It is one of the most obvious combinations of East and West. At its best it is able to compete with the world's best; at its most boring, it is **anything** *with a slice of pineapple! This recipe makes good use of an older, large bird, and uses the juice—not a slice!*

INGREDIENTS

Chicken

6 cloves	GARLIC
1	WHOLE CHICKEN (4 1/2–5 lb.)

Pineapple Curry Sauce

1 teaspoon	LIGHT OLIVE OIL
3/4 cup	FINELY DICED SWEET ONION
1 Tablespoon	GOOD MADRAS CURRY POWDER
1 Tablespoon	PEELED AND GRATED GINGERROOT
2 large cloves	GARLIC, peeled, bashed, and finely chopped
3/4 cup	LOW-SODIUM CHICKEN OR VEGETABLE STOCK (pp. 222, 225)
1/3 cup	FROZEN PINEAPPLE JUICE CONCENTRATE
1/4 cup	YOGURT CHEESE (p. 38, n. 10)
1/2 teaspoon	COCONUT EXTRACT (p. 33, n. 26)
1 Tablespoon	THAI FISH SAUCE (p. 32, n. 21)
1 Tablespoon	CORNSTARCH

BEFORE YOU COOK:

Peel and crush garlic. Wash chicken, dry with paper towels. Finely dice onion, grate the ginger. Measure remaining ingredients.

COOKING METHOD

To Prepare the Chicken:

1. Preheat the oven to 350°F.
2. Put the garlic into the cavity of the chicken. Turn the chicken breast down on a plate so that the seasonings falls against the inside of the breast. Insert a vertical poultry roaster (see p. 41, n. 5) into the chicken and stand upright. Tie the legs together with cotton string and tuck

the wings behind the breast. (If you don't have a vertical roster, lay the chicken on a rack in a roasting pan.)

3. Whichever roasting method you are using, pour 1 1/2 cups of warm water into the bottom of the baking dish. Bake in the preheated oven for 1 to 1 1/2 hours, or until the chicken reaches 140°F in the thickest part of the thigh. (The chicken in the roasting pan may take an extra 10 mins.) Remove from the oven and set aside for 10 minutes. The final internal temperature should be 160°F.

To Prepare the Sauce:

1. Warm the oil in a medium saucepan over medium heat. Sauté the onion and curry power until the onion is soft and translucent, about 5 minutes. Stir in the ginger and garlic, and cook for 3 more minutes. Add the stock and pineapple juice concentrate, stirring to incorporate. Cook for an additional 3 minutes. Strain the sauce through a sieve into a small saucepan using the back of a spoon.

2. Whisk together the yogurt cheese, coconut extract, cornstarch, and Thai fish sauce in a 2-cup glass measuring cup. Pour a little of the hot pineapple sauce into the yogurt mixture and stir to warm the yogurt cheese. Add the "tempered" yogurt cheese to the sauce and whisk until smooth. Cover and set aside to keep warm (it should not boil).

To Assemble the Dish:

1. Remove the chicken from the roasting pan and pour the cooking juices into a fat strainer. Remove and discard the skin. Cut the legs and breast meat away from the carcass. Put aside 1 breast for another meal. Slice the meat from the remaining breast and legs and arrange on a warmed plate. Cover and keep warm.

2. Pour the defatted pan juices into a small saucepan. Allow to cool for a minute, then stir into the curry sauce. Arrange slices of chicken on a warmed plate and spoon curry sauce over the meat. Serve Vegetable Stir-Fry alongside.

NUTRITIONAL ANALYSIS

Per serving: 297 calories, 44 g protein, 12 g carbohydrate, 8 g fat, 2 g saturated fat, 6% calories from saturated fat, 1 g dietary fiber

AT A GLANCE
(FOR SKILLED COOKS IN A HURRY)

Season chicken with garlic inside. Truss and roast on vertical stand or on trivet at 350°F for 60–90 minutes until 140°F at the thigh. Set and test after 10 minutes should be 160°F. *Sauce:* Warm oil. Sauté onion and curry powder. Add ginger and garlic. Sauté with Thai fish sauce. Add hot pineapple carefully to yogurt. Whisk smooth. Slice the bird. Coat with sauce.

Chicken and Pineapple Adobo

SERVES 4

This is a simple stovetop solution to the common chicken stew. It's an all-in-one dish that requires very little of your time, yet delivers a wonderful range of tastes, textures, and aromas.

INGREDIENTS

1 teaspoon	NONAROMATIC OLIVE OIL
1 Tablespoon	LEMON JUICE
4	MEDIUM CHICKEN THIGHS, skinned and trimmed of fat
1/8 tsp. + 1/4 tsp.	SALT
1/4 teaspoon	FRESHLY GROUND BLACK PEPPER
1	SMALL RED PEPPER
1	SMALL GREEN PEPPER
2 cloves	GARLIC
2 cups	LOW-SODIUM CHICKEN STOCK (p. 225)
2	TURKISH BAY LEAVES
2 cups	FRESH PINEAPPLE CHUNKS
1 (16-oz. can)	GREAT NORTHERN BEANS
2	ROMA TOMATOES
1 Tablespoon	CHOPPED FRESH PARSLEY
1/4 cup	LIME JUICE
2 teaspoon	ARROWROOT, plus 4 teaspoons water (slurry)

BEFORE YOU COOK:

Cut the peppers into 1-inch squares; crush the garlic; drain and rinse the canned beans. Cut the tomatoes in 1-inch chunks. Chop the parsley. Measure remaining ingredients.

COOKING METHOD

1. Heat the oil and lemon juice in a large skillet on medium high. Season the chicken with 1/8 teaspoon each of salt and pepper. Fry one side for 2 minutes or until browned. Reduce heat to medium low, and turn the chicken. Add the pepper pieces and garlic, and sauté 2 more minutes, being careful not to brown the garlic.

2. Pour stock into the pan, add bay leaves, cover, and simmer for 20 minutes. Add pineapple and beans, and simmer 10 minutes more. Stir in tomato chunks, parsley, 2 tablespoons of lime juice, 1/4 teaspoon salt, and 1/8 teaspoon pepper. Taste, and add more lime juice if you like (3 tablespoons was right for me, and it should be slightly sour). Pour in the slurry, stirring

constantly until the liquid thickens, less than 30 seconds; remove bay leaves. This is another all-in-one dish.

NUTRITIONAL ANALYSIS

Per serving: 295 calories, 33 g carbohydrate, 9 g fat, 2 g saturated fat, 7% calories from saturated fat, 447 mg sodium, 7 g dietary fiber

AT A GLANCE
(FOR SKILLED COOKS IN A HURRY)

Heat oil and lemon juice; sauté seasoned chicken to brown (2 mins. plus). Reduce heat, turn, add peppers and garlic; sauté another 2 minutes. Add stock, bay leaves, cover, and simmer 20 minutes. Add pineapple and beans for 10 minutes, then add tomato, parsley, lime juice (taste as you go). Add slurry to thicken. Serve.

Brunswick Stew

*If I had to make a choice, this would be my pick as the best regional stew in North America. Its roots go all the way back to the early trappers, and no doubt it has changed, but the beans, corn, and bacon—along with their trapped critter meats—must have been great when spooned out of the cast iron camp kettle onto enamel plates. Ahhhh, such **was** the life—or was it?*

INGREDIENTS

3 1/2 pound	FRYING CHICKEN (or 2 boneless, skinless breasts and 2 hindquarters)
1 teaspoon	NONAROMATIC OLIVE OIL, divided
1 large	SWEET ONION (generous 2 c.)
3 ribs	CELERY (1 1/2 c.)
3 ounces	CANADIAN BACON
1	RED BELL PEPPER
2 cups	CANNED, CRUSHED TOMATOES
1 cup	LOW-SODIUM CHICKEN STOCK (p. 225)
1 Tablespoon	WORCESTERSHIRE SAUCE
1/4 teaspoon	CAYENNE PEPPER
2 cups	FROZEN CORN KERNELS
1 cup	FROZEN BABY LIMA BEANS
1 Tablespoon	ARROWROOT mixed with
2 Tablespoons	STOCK OR WATER (slurry)
1/4 cup	CHOPPED FRESH PARSLEY
1/4 cup	CHOPPED FRESH BASIL

BEFORE YOU COOK:

Rinse chicken pieces and dry on paper towel. Cut sweet onion in 1-inch dice. Cut celery, red pepper, and Canadian bacon into 1/4-inch slices. Measure remaining ingredients.

COOKING METHOD

1. If you are using a whole chicken, cut off the legs with the thighs and the breasts. Use the carcass and wings for stock. Remove the skin from all the pieces. Separate the legs from the thighs and bone the thigh, leaving the bone in the leg. Remove the skin and bone from the breast pieces. Bones, fat, and skin will all help to make a flavorful stock. Cut the meat into 1 1/2-inch chunks.

2. Heat 1/2 teaspoon of the oil in a 10 1/2-inch chef's pan on medium high. Sauté the onion 3 minutes or until starting to turn translucent. Add the celery, Canadian bacon, and red bell

pepper and cook 3 more minutes. Remove to a plate and without washing the pan, add the remaining 1/2 teaspoon oil and heat. When the pan is nice and hot, toss in the thigh meat and legs to brown 2 minutes. Add the breast meat and brown 1 to 2 minutes more.

3. Pour in the tomatoes, stock, and Worcestershire sauce. Add the cooked vegetables/Canadian bacon mix and cayenne. Bring to a boil, reduce the heat, cover, and simmer 35 minutes or until the chicken is tender. Add the lima beans and corn and cook 12 minutes more or until the beans are tender. Stir in the slurry and heat to thicken. Add the parsley and basil, and you are ready to serve.

NUTRITIONAL ANALYSIS

Per serving: 260 calories, 21 g carbohydrate, 6 g fat, 2 g saturated fat, 7% calories from saturated fat, 362 mg sodium, 3 g dietary fiber

AT A GLANCE
(FOR SKILLED COOKS IN A HURRY)

Cut chicken into pan pieces. Heat oil. Sauté onion. Add celery, bacon, bell pepper. Sauté 3 minutes. Remove to plate. Heat pan to high. Sauté chicken pieces to brown (legs first, then breast). Add tomato, stock, Worcestershire sauce, and cooked vegetables. Cover, simmer 35 minutes until tender. Add lima beans and corn for additional 12 minutes. Thicken. Dust with parsley and basil. Serve.

St. Augustine Perlow

SERVES 6

"Perlow" is the southern way of saying Pilau, and if anyone should know how to fix it, it's the folks from the oldest city in North America—St. Augustine in Florida. They brought their great culinary traditions with them, and they cultivated an extraordinary pepper—the datil. To make this dish, you may wish to track it down (see Buying, p. 34, n. 28).

INGREDIENTS

1 teaspoon	NONAROMATIC OLIVE OIL
1 cup	FINELY CHOPPED ONION
1 clove	GARLIC
1/4 pound	CANADIAN BACON
1	LARGE RED BELL PEPPER
3/4 cup	CELERY
4	ROMA TOMATOES
1 teaspoon	MILD CHILI POWDER
1/4 teaspoon	THYME
pinch	CLOVES
1/4 teaspoon	DATIL CHILI POWDER or cayenne pepper
1 teaspoon	SALT
1 cup	LONG-GRAIN WHITE RICE
2 cups	LOW-SODIUM CHICKEN STOCK (p. 225)
1/2	COOKED CHICKEN BREAST (4 oz.)
2	COOKED CHICKEN THIGHS
15	LARGE BLACK PITTED OLIVES
2 Tablespoons	CHOPPED PARSLEY

BEFORE YOU COOK:

Crush garlic. Cut bacon, celery, bell pepper, and tomatoes into 1/2-inch dice. Wash the rice and drain. Bone and skin the cooked chicken pieces. Cut in roughly 1-inch pieces. Chop parsley.

COOKING METHOD

1. Preheat the oven to 450°F. Heat the oil in a large skillet or chef's pan on medium high. Sauté the onion 2 minutes or until it starts to wilt. Add the garlic and cook 1 minute more. Stir in the bacon, bell pepper, tomatoes, celery, chili powder, thyme, cloves, datil (or cayenne), and salt. Cook, stirring, 5 minutes more. Stir in the rice and pour the stock over all. Bake, uncovered, in the preheated oven 20 minutes or until the rice is tender and fluffy.

2. Add the chicken and olives, mix, and return to the oven for 6 more minutes to heat through. Serve on hot plates scattered with fresh parsley.

NUTRITIONAL ANALYSIS

Per serving: 275 calories, 33 g carbohydrate, 7 g fat, 2 g saturated fat, 7% calories from saturated fat, 812 mg sodium, 3 g dietary fiber

AT A GLANCE
(FOR SKILLED COOKS IN A HURRY)

Preheat oven to 450°F. Heat oil in skillet. Sauté onion. Add garlic. Stir in bacon, celery, bell pepper, tomato, chili powder, thyme, cloves, datil (or cayenne), and salt. Stir 5 minutes. Add rice. Pour in stock. Bake 20 minutes. Add chicken and olives. Heat in oven 6 to 10 minutes. Serve with parsley.

Chicken Enchiladas

*I know people who will drive for untold miles to eat a **specific** enchilada. We did too—all the way to San Antonio, Texas, and it was a triumph. At one time in my "gourmet" past life, I **loved** the fine French pancakes (crepes) filled with a dense creamy combination of seafood. It's that same feeling I get from a really good enchilada, and it doesn't **have** to be overrich or overlarge to do the trick. Try this one from San Antonio?*

INGREDIENTS

Sauce

1/2 teaspoon	NONAROMATIC OLIVE OIL
1/2 cup	ROUGHLY CHOPPED ONIONS
1 clove	GARLIC
1	JALAPENO CHILI
1/4 teaspoon	CAYENNE PEPPER (optional)
1 teaspoon	GROUND CUMIN
1 pound	ROMA TOMATOES
1 (10 3/4 oz. can)	TOMATO PUREE
1 teaspoon	DRIED OREGANO
1 1/2 cups	LOW-SODIUM CHICKEN STOCK (p. 225)

Filling

8 ounces	BONED, SKIN-ON CHICKEN BREAST
1 cup	LOW-SODIUM CHICKEN STOCK (p. 225)
1/2 cup	LOW-FAT COTTAGE CHEESE
1/4 cup	LOW-FAT YOGURT
2 Tablespoons	CHOPPED CILANTRO
2 teaspoons	CORNSTARCH
4	WHOLE CANNED MILD GREEN CHILIES
1/4 cup	FINELY CHOPPED ONION
8	5-INCH FLOUR TORTILLAS (cut larger ones to size)
1/2 cup	LOW-FAT MONTEREY JACK CHEESE

BEFORE YOU COOK:

Roughly chop onion (1/2 c.). Finely chop onion (1/4 c.). Crush garlic. Seed and chop jalapeno. Roughly chop tomatoes. Cut canned green chilies in 1/2-inch strips.

COOKING METHOD

1. Preheat the oven to 350°F. Heat oil in a pan and sauté 1/2 cup onion for 2 minutes. Add garlic, jalapeno, cayenne, and cumin, and cook 2 minutes. Stir in tomatoes, tomato puree, and oregano. Whip in blender or processor, return to pan, and add chicken stock. Bring to a boil; then simmer 20 minutes.

2. Place chicken breast, skin side up, in small skillet. Add stock and cover with a piece of waxed paper cut to size. Bring to a boil, reduce heat, and poach gently 20 minutes. Cool, remove skin, and cut across the grain in thin slices. It may still be a little pink but will finish cooking with the enchiladas.

3. Blend or process cottage cheese until smooth. Add yogurt, cilantro, and cornstarch, and pulse to mix.

4. Spoon a little sauce into a 9-inch x 13-inch baking dish. Dip a tortilla in the sauce and lay on a plate. Spread a tablespoon of the cottage cheese mixture down the center. Lay pieces of chicken and green chilies on top and sprinkle with onion. Roll and lay in the baking dish. Repeat for all tortillas. Cover with remaining sauce, scatter cheese on top, and bake 20 minutes or until heated through.

NUTRITIONAL ANALYSIS

Per serving: 361 calories, 45 g carbohydrate, 9 g fat, 3 g saturated fat, 7% calories from saturated fat, 970 mg sodium, 6 g dietary fiber

AT A GLANCE
(FOR SKILLED COOKS IN A HURRY)

Preheat oven 350°F. Heat oil and sauté onion. Add garlic, jalapeno, cayenne, and cumin. Cook 2 minutes. Stir in tomato, puree, and oregano. Whiz in blender or processor and return to pan. Add stock, boil, and simmer 20 minutes. Put chicken breast in small skillet. Add stock. Cover with waxed paper. Boil then reduce heat. Poach 20 minutes. Cool. Slice across grain thinly. Blend cheese until smooth. Add yogurt, cilantro, and cornstarch. Mix well. Spoon "red" sauce into small baking dish (9 x 13-in.). Coat tortilla with same sauce. Lay on plate. Add a spoonful "white" sauce. Top chicken and chilies with onion. Roll up. Lay side by side. Scatter cheese. Bake 20 minutes. Serve.

Jambalaya

*I use an acronym F.A.B.I.S. that spells out as **fresh and best in season.** It underlines the source of true "regionality." If certain ingredients are truly **local,** they will all be available during one month or so in a specific location. That's the only way it can be called a 'regional cuisine.' Just because a number of Scots settled in the northeast U.S.A. doesn't make pickled black walnut and beef stew a regional dish. All this to say how much I celebrate this southern specialty. Shrimp, rice, bell peppers, ham, celery, sausage—what a wonderful dish.*

INGREDIENTS

2 cups	LOW-SODIUM CHICKEN STOCK (p. 225)
1/2 pound	MEDIUM RAW SHRIMP, peeled and deveined
1 cup	LONG-GRAIN WHITE RICE
1/4 teaspoon	SALT
3	BAY LEAVES
1 1/2 teaspoon	NONAROMATIC OLIVE OIL, divided
3	SPICY LOW-FAT CHICKEN SAUSAGES (12 oz.)
1 large	SWEET ONION, cut in half and sliced stem to root
4 cloves	GARLIC, bashed and chopped
1 Tablespoon	TOMATO PASTE
1 large	RED BELL PEPPER, cut in 1 1/2-inch strips
3 ounces	CANADIAN BACON, cut in 1 1/2-inch strips
1 large	RIB CELERY, cut in 1 1/2-inch strips
1/4 teaspoon	CAYENNE PEPPER
1/4 teaspoon	THYME
pinch	CLOVES
8	ROMA TOMATOES, peeled, seeded, chopped or one 28-ounce can diced tomatoes in juice
1/4 cup	CHOPPED PARSLEY

BEFORE YOU COOK:

Peel and devein shrimp. Finely slice onion. Crush garlic. Cut the bell pepper, Canadian bacon, and celery into 1 1/2 inch strips. Seed and chop tomatoes (or use canned). Chop parsley.

COOKING METHOD

1. Bring the stock to a boil in a medium saucepan. Drop the shrimp in and cook 2 minutes. Remove shrimp and set aside. Measure the stock and add water to make 2 cups. Add the rice,

salt, and bay leaves and cook gently 15 minutes or until tender and the liquid is gone. Set aside. Heat 1 teaspoon of the oil in a 10 1/2-inch chef's pan and fry the sausages, turning often, 10 minutes on medium high or until nearly done. Cut in rounds and set aside.

2. Pour the remaining 1/2 teaspoon oil into the pan and shallow fry the onion until it turns translucent, 3–4 minutes. Add the garlic and tomato paste and continue cooking until the paste darkens (8–10 mins.). Now toss in the celery, red pepper, and Canadian bacon and cook until the vegetables are crisp but tender. Season with cayenne, thyme, and cloves. Stir in the tomatoes, parsley, and reserved shrimp and cook until just heated through. Add the rice and mix well.

NUTRITIONAL ANALYSIS

Per serving: 314 calories, 23 g protein, 38 g carbohydrate, 8 g fat, 2 g saturated fat, 5% calories from saturated fat, 666 mg sodium, 3 g fiber

AT A GLANCE
(FOR SKILLED COOKS IN A HURRY)

Boil stock. Add peeled shrimp. Cook 2 minutes. Remove to plate. Use 2 cups water/stock to cook rice. Add salt and bay leaves. Boil. Reduce and cook 15 minutes to absorb liquid. Heat oil in skillet. Sauté sausages (10 mins.). Cut in rounds. Add oil and sauté onion. Add garlic and tomato paste. Stir to darken. Add celery, pepper, bacon—cook till crisp. Season with cayenne, thyme, and cloves. Add tomatoes, parsley, and cooked shrimp. Add rice and fold in well.

Roast Duck Breasts

Not all ducks are ducklings, but then not all ducklings are tender. We've long since decided to treat the breast differently from the less tender leg and thigh meat. It works wonderfully well, so here goes with one "duckling" and three recipes—all of which make wonderful, flavorsome, and nourishing meals for two.

INGREDIENTS

4 1/2 pounds	DUCKLING
1 teaspoon	OLIVE OIL
season	SALT
season	WHITE PEPPER

BEFORE YOU COOK:

Remove the breasts, leaving enough skin and fat to cover the breast meat; each should weigh 6 to 7 ounces. At the same time, remove the legs and thighs for later use. Chop up the carcass to be used as Duck Stock (see p. 224).

COOKING METHOD

1. Preheat the oven to 375°F. Add oil to pan (brush or spray on).
2. Season the breasts, especially the cut surfaces, with salt and white pepper. Lay skin side up on a rack in a baking pan and roast for 25 minutes or until the internal temperature reaches 170°F for pale pink.
3. When done, let them rest so the juices set before carving. Remove skin and fat. We prefer to serve either whole or sliced across the grain into about twelve thin pieces.
4. Red currant jelly goes well, and a simple orange and butter lettuce salad is tremendous!

NUTRITIONAL ANALYSIS

Per serving: 179 calories, 31 g protein, 0 g carbohydrates, 5 g fat, 1 g saturated fat, 421 mg sodium, 11 mg calcium, 5 mg iron, 17 RE Vitamin A, 4 mg Vitamin C, 1 mg Vitamin E, 0 g fiber

AT A GLANCE
(FOR SKILLED COOKS IN A HURRY)

Remove breasts, trim, and use carcass for stock. Preheat oven to 375°F. Roast for 25 minutes (pink) internal temperature 170°F. Set juices. Serve whole or carve.

Braised Legs and Thighs of Duckling

SERVES 2-4

For reasons explained on page 152, we prefer to separate the breast and the leg/thigh meat and use different methods of cooking. This also helps to deal with the quite large amounts of fat if a duck is roasted whole. Roast duck fat is so delicious that it can be irresistible until it shows up on the scales or a lab report! So, here goes with a great dish that doesn't show up on either.

INGREDIENTS

season	SALT and WHITE PEPPER
14 ounces	LEG/THIGH FROM 4 1/2-LB. DUCKLING (see p. 152)
2 cups	FINELY CHOPPED SWEET ONION
1 1/2 cups	DICED GREEN PEPPERS (or Poblanos*)
10 ounces	PINEAPPLE, cut in 1-inch wedges
1 1/2 cups	DUCK STOCK (see p. 224)
2 cups	FROZEN GREEN PEAS
1 Tablespoon	CORNSTARCH

BEFORE YOU COOK:

Trim the skin and excess fat from leg/thigh. Fine-chop the onion; seed and dice peppers. (*If Poblanos are used, cut, flatten, and broil the hard outer skin; peel and then dice). Dice pineapple. Skim duck stock. Measure remaining ingredients.

COOKING METHOD

1. Preheat the oven to 375°F. Season the duck meat. Lay in a baking pan. Surround the duck pieces with the onion and peppers. Roast, fat side up, for 25 minutes.
2. Turn the roasted duck and vegetables into a medium saucepan. Add the pineapple and stock.
3. Simmer gently to blend the flavors.
4. Thicken the sauce with cornstarch mixed to a cream with cold water. Add frozen peas and bring to a boil for 1 full minute. Adjust seasoning and serve.

NUTRITIONAL ANALYSIS

Per serving: 429 calories, 33 g protein, 57 g carbohydrates, 8 g fat, 3 g saturated fat, 584 mg sodium, 62 mg calcium, 5 mg iron, 149 RE Vitamin A, 71 mg Vitamin C, 2 mg Vitamin E, 13 g fiber

AT A GLANCE
(FOR SKILLED COOKS IN A HURRY)

Roast duck pieces at 375°F with onion and peppers for 25 minutes. Turn into saucepan and add pineapple. Simmer. Thicken with cornstarch. Add peas and boil to clear. Serve.

Duck Breasts and Pineapple Stir-Fry

SERVES 2

It is our personal preference to slightly undercook a roast to get the meat for a stir-fry. Too often meat cooked from raw becomes tough, rubbery, and obviously shrunken when treated classically. When it isn't, then it can be undercooked! We get the best of all worlds by adding the partially cooked meat at the end, to heat through, and usually an extra meal too!

INGREDIENTS

10–12 ounces	ROASTED DUCK BREASTS (see p. 152)
1 Tablespoon	OLIVE OIL
1/4 teaspoon	SESAME SEED OIL
1 Tablespoon	FINELY SLICED GINGERROOT
2 cloves	GARLIC, crushed
8-ounce can	SLICED WATER CHESTNUTS
1/4 pound	SNOW PEAS (fresh)
2/3 cup	FRESH PINEAPPLE
1–2 Tablespoons	LOW SODIUM SOY SAUCE
1 cup	DUCK STOCK (see p. 224)
2 teaspoons	ARROWROOT or cornstarch

BEFORE YOU COOK:

Slice duck into 1/4-inch thick pieces. Slice ginger and crush garlic. Measure oils and mix. Drain water chestnuts. Top 'n' tail snow peas. Slice and dice pineapple. Measure remaining ingredients. Warm the duck stock.

COOKING METHOD

1. Heat a large skillet or wok on medium-high heat. Add mixed oils.
2. Add ginger and garlic. Sauté 1 minute. Add water chestnuts, snow peas, and pineapple. Toss to heat through, 2 minutes.
3. Add soy sauce to your taste. Toss well and add the duck breast. Pour in the stock. Cover.
4. Make a light cream by combining the arrowroot or cornstarch to 1 tablespoon of water. Stir into the hot stock to thicken and clear, 30 seconds.
5. Serve with steamed rice (see p. 93).

NUTRITIONAL ANALYSIS

Per serving: 334 calories, 24 g protein, 21 g carbohydrates, 17 g saturated fat*, 546 mg sodium, 59 mg calcium, 4 mg iron, 33 RE Vitamin A, 44 mg Vitamin C, 3 mg Vitamin E, 4 g fiber

Our software doesn't allow for the fat we trimmed, so please know that the actual fat is less!

AT A GLANCE
(FOR SKILLED COOKS IN A HURRY)

Slice duck 1/4-inch. Sauté ginger and garlic. Add chestnuts, snow peas, and pineapple. Toss 2 minutes. Add soy sauce and duck stock. Boil, thicken with starch, and serve with rice.

Italian Meat Sauce with Turkey

MAKES 56 OZ. (OR 8 SERVINGS)

*It is no surprise to me that the most popular ethnic food style in the United States is Italian. As a nation, Italy has a wonderfully wide variety of regional styles best suited to its range of climates. Of all the regions, I prefer Regis Emelia and the city of Bologna, from which the world famous meat sauce originated—***Salsa Bolognaise.*** My task in life is to simplify and to some extent lessen the health risks of such great dishes yet without doing damage to the original genus! Here goes, using the now widely available ground turkey as the meat base instead of beef. We make up a large batch and freeze it in four pouches, each serving two. It's our own "too-tired-to-cook" dish when we've exceeded our speed limit for the day!*

INGREDIENTS

1 Tbsp. + 2 tsps.	OLIVE OIL
1 pound	FRESHLY GROUND TURKEY
1/2 pound	ONION
3	GARLIC CLOVES
3 Tablespoons	TOMATO PASTE
1 16-ounce can	CHOPPED TOMATOES (see p. 29, n. 1)
2 cups	CHICKEN STOCK
1 cup	DE-ALCOHOLIZED WHITE WINE
1 Tablespoon	HERBS OF PROVENCE
1 pound	PASTA (type is your choice) (2 oz. per person)
1 Tablespoon	ARROWROOT
3 cups	LEAF SPINACH

BEFORE YOU COOK:

Crush garlic. Finely slice the spinach and then lightly chop to reduce the leaf length to a short strand. Finely chop the onion. Measure remaining ingredients.

COOKING METHOD

1. In a large skillet (10–12 in. diameter) heat 1 Tablespoon of the oil until very hot (350–375°F). Add ground turkey a spoon at a time and scatter over hot surface to brown and to some extent evaporate surplus juices—takes about 10 minutes. Turn out into a bowl.
2. Add the remaining 2 teaspoons oil to the unwashed pan. Add chopped onion. Sauté until just turning color, then add crushed garlic.

3. Stir in the tomato paste well and cook until the paste darkens. Add the chopped tomatoes, chicken stock, white wine, and herbs. Stir well. Return the turkey to the pan. Cover and simmer for 10 minutes.

4. Meanwhile cook your pasta according to packet instructions, about 11–12 minutes if dried; 4–8 minutes, if fresh.

5. Moisten the arrowroot (or cornstarch) with a little wine and thicken the sauce (see Culinary Techniques, p. 37, n. 7). Stir in the sliced spinach (this is not in the classic ingredient, but I happen to like it!). It cooks instantly.

6. Serve over pasta and, please, enjoy it!

NUTRITIONAL ANALYSIS

Per serving: 347 calories, 21 g protein, 49 g carbohydrates, 8 g fat, 2 g saturated fat, 200 mg sodium, 40 mg calcium, 4 mg iron, 87 RE Vitamin A, 14 mg Vitamin C, 1 mg Vitamin E, 4 g fiber

AT A GLANCE
(FOR SKILLED COOKS IN A HURRY)

Brown turkey well (10 mins.). Turn out. Sauté onion. Add garlic. Cook tomato paste to darken. Add chopped tomatoes, chicken stock, wine, and herbs. Return turkey to sauce. Simmer 10 minutes. Cook pasta and drain. Thicken sauce. Add spinach. Coat pasta to serve.

Turkey Potpie

I found this idea in the oldest inn in the United States in upper New York State and loved both the place and the concept of the cheese biscuit instead of the standard pastry crust. I halved the biscuit quantity and used my parsnip "velvet" sauce to replace their very rich turkey gravy. It works really well and has become one of our favorites for the day after Thanksgiving.

INGREDIENTS

Pie Filling

1 teaspoon	NONAROMATIC OLIVE OIL
1/2	SWEET ONION (1 c.)
2	CARROTS (1 c.)
2	TURNIPS (1 c.)
2	SMALL PARSNIPS (1/2 c.)
1 1/2 cups	HOMEMADE TURKEY or low-sodium chicken stock (p. 225)
1/8 teaspoon	PEPPER
1 pound	BROCCOLI
2 1/2 cups	COOKED TURKEY (2/3 dark and 1/3 white meat)

Sauce

3/4 pound	PARSNIPS
1 cup	EVAPORATED SKIM MILK
1/4 teaspoon	SALT

Cheese Biscuits *(Whole wheat phyllo can be used to reduce both fat and carbs: p. 34, n. 33.)*

1 cup	ALL-PURPOSE FLOUR
1 cup	CAKE FLOUR
1 Tablespoon	SUGAR
1 1/2 teaspoons	BAKING POWDER
1/2 teaspoon	BAKING SODA
1/4 teaspoon	SALT
1 1/2 Tablespoons	COLD, HARD BUTTER
3/4 cup	BUTTERMILK
1 Tablespoon	NONAROMATIC OLIVE OIL
1/4 cup	GRATED LOW-FAT SHARP CHEDDAR CHEESE
1 Tablespoon	LOW-FAT MILK (to brush on top)

BEFORE YOU COOK:

Cut the onion into 1/4-inch dice. Cut the carrot, turnip, and parsnip into 1/2-inch dice. Cut the cooked turkey into 1/2-inch dice (remove all fat/skin). **Sauce:** cut parsnip, rough chop, and steam until very tender. **Biscuit:** cut butter into 1/4-inch pieces. Keep chilled. Measure remaining ingredients.

COOKING METHOD

1. Heat the oil in a chef's pan or skillet on medium high. Sauté the onions, carrots, turnips, and parsnips on medium heat 3 minutes. Pour in the stock and season with salt and pepper. Bring to a boil, reduce the heat, cover, and simmer until the vegetables are tender, about 6 minutes.
2. Whiz the steamed parsnips in a blender with a little of the evaporated milk until smooth, about 2 minutes. Add the rest of the milk and the salt and whiz until smooth and velvety, another 30 seconds.
3. Preheat the oven to 425°F. Coat a baking sheet with pan spray. Whisk together the flours, sugar, baking powder, soda, and salt in a bowl or combine in a processor.
4. Scatter the pieces of margarine over the top and cut in with 2 knives or pulse 2 or 3 times in the processor. Make a well in the center of the dry ingredients and pour in the buttermilk and oil. Stir with a fork just until blended, or pulse 2 or 3 times in the processor.
5. Knead the dough very lightly on a floured board. Pat or roll out about 1/2 inch thick and cut into four large 3-inch biscuits. Place on the prepared baking sheet, brush with milk, dust with cheese, and bake 15 minutes or until golden.
6. While the biscuits are baking, lay the broccoli on the simmering vegetables and cook until tender, 6 minutes or until tender but still bright green. Stir in the turkey and parsnip sauce and heat through.
7. Biscuits by the nature of their chemistry are high in calories and fat. To fit into your meal plan, make a whole recipe, cut the tops off four to use in the recipe, and save the bottoms and extra biscuit to toast for breakfast. Spoon the turkey mixture into four hot soup plates and lay the biscuit halves on top.

NUTRITIONAL ANALYSIS

Per serving: 485 calories, 39 g protein, 60 g carbohydrate, 10 g fat, 4 g saturated fat, 1% calories from saturated fat, 739 mg sodium, 10 g dietary fiber (see note above about phyllo)

AT A GLANCE
(FOR SKILLED COOKS IN A HURRY)

Heat oil. Sauté onion, carrot, turnip, and parsnip for 3 minutes. Add stock. Season. Boil, reduce, cover, and simmer until tender (6 mins.). *Sauce:* whiz steamed parsnips in blender with 1/4 cup evaporated milk (2–7 mins.). Add remaining milk and salt. Whiz until "velvet." *Biscuits:* oven 425°F. Oil tray. Whisk all dry ingredients. Cut in the butter. Make a well and add liquids. Fork lightly to combine. Kneed lightly. Roll out 1/2 inch thick. Cut out 2-inch round biscuits. Brush with milk and dust with cheese. Bake 15 minutes. During baking, add broccoli and turkey to vegetables for 6 minutes. Add sauce (taste for seasoning). Serve in bowl topped with half a biscuit.

Roasted Young Chicken   SERVES 4

In the restless search for convenience, consumers have discovered the spit-roasted chicken at our supermarkets. We submit a simple alternative that saves money, sodium, and saturated fats. It takes time, which to our **taste** *is well worth it!*

INGREDIENTS

3 pounds	YOUNG "FRYER" CHICKEN (organic or your choice)
1 Tablespoon	OLIVE OIL
season	SALT
season	WHITE PEPPER
garnish	PAPRIKA
garnish	PARSLEY, fine chopped
1/4 cup	RED CURRANT JELLY (optional)

BEFORE YOU COOK:

Remove chicken wrapper. Rinse under cold running water. Dry on paper towels.

COOKING METHOD

1. Preheat the oven to 375° or 350°F for convection.
2. Brush olive oil over dry chicken skin. Season lightly all over with salt and pepper. Place the chicken on its side on a wire rack in a roasting pan. Roast in the preheated oven for 20 minutes.
3. Turn to other side and continue roasting for another 20 minutes. Turn breast side up for the last 20 minutes of roasting. That's 1 hour of total cooking time.
4. Remove the chicken when the internal temperature in the thigh is 170°F. Cover with a tent of aluminum foil to retain heat. The internal temperature will rise to 180°F as it sits.
5. The red currant jelly always goes well!

NUTRITIONAL ANALYSIS

Per serving: 386 calories, 49 g protein, 13 g carbohydrates, 14 g fat, 3 g saturated fat, 448 mg sodium, 25 mg calcium, 1 mg iron, 191 RE Vitamin A, 0 mg Vitamin C, 1 mg Vitamin E, 0 g fiber

AT A GLANCE
(FOR SKILLED COOKS IN A HURRY)

Wash, dry, oil, and season. Oven at 375°F or 350°F convection. Roast 20 minutes on either side—finish breast up. Total 60 minutes. Internal temperature 170°F. Stand, covered, 10 minutes. Carve.

Basque-style Skillet Stewed Chicken

A wide 11-inch diameter, 3-inch deep skillet complete with a lid is one of our most treasured pieces of kitchen equipment. It makes a perfect skillet stew for up to six people—much better than a saucepan. That old electric fry pan idea was a good one! Here is our take on the famous Basque country dish.

INGREDIENTS

2 teaspoons	OLIVE OIL, divided
2 pounds*	CHICKEN THIGHS
1 medium	SWEET ONION, finely sliced
2	GARLIC CLOVES, crushed
1 large	SWEET RED BELL PEPPER
2 medium	TOMATOES
2 Tablespoons	HERBS OF PROVENCE
1 teaspoon	SALT
1 cup	VEGETABLE STOCK (p. 222)
1 Tablespoon	CORNSTARCH (mixed with water)
1 Tablespoon	PARSLEY
2 cups tightly packed	BABY SPINACH LEAVES
Optional	MUSHROOMS, (p. 31, n. 13)

BEFORE YOU COOK:

Trim skin and fat from thighs (*reduces weight by 8 oz.) and discard. Wash and dry. *Finely* slice onion, pepper, and tomatoes (no need to remove skins if finely sliced). Measure remaining ingredients.

COOKING METHOD

1. Heat large skillet or saucepan on medium high (300°F). Add 1 teaspoon oil.
2. Add thighs, round side down, for 5 minutes to brown, with the lid on.
3. Remove thighs and reheat pan until sizzle stops. Add 1 teaspoon of the oil, heat, and add the onion. Fry for 2 minutes, add garlic and cook, stirring for 2 more minutes. Stir in the red peppers. Return the thighs to the pan cut side down. Spoon the vegetables over the top and cook 10 minutes with the lid on.

4. Smother with sliced tomatoes and sprinkle with Herbs of Provence and 1/4 teaspoon of the salt. Pour in the vegetable stock, replace lid, and simmer 10 minutes. The chicken has now been cooked 25 minutes and should be at 180°F.
5. Remove chicken and cut away the bones. Return the meat to the skillet.
6. Stir in the cornstarch cream to thicken. Test for seasoning (there is 3/4 tsp. salt waiting to be used!). Add parsley and optional mushrooms. Serve hot over fresh, raw, baby spinach leaves.

NUTRITIONAL ANALYSIS

Per serving: 241 calories, 30 g protein, 12 g carbohydrates, 8 g fat, 2 g saturated fat, 721 mg sodium, 50 calcium, 3 mg iron, 321 RE Vitamin A, 81 mg Vitamin C, 2 mg Vitamin E, 4 g fiber

AT A GLANCE
(FOR SKILLED COOKS IN A HURRY)

Trim off fat/skin and sauté round side down 5 minutes, covered. Remove and add oil. Sauté onion and garlic. Add sweet peppers. Return thighs and smother with tomatoes, herbs, and salt. 10 minutes. Add vegetable stock, 10 minutes. Bone and return meat. Thicken. Add parsley and serve.

Chicken Stir-Fry, Thai Style

The Thai people have learned over centuries to make very good use of naturally growing aromats—ginger, garlic, lemon grass, coconut, and even their famed fish sauce. All go together brilliantly in this dish. It may even spur you on to your own creations.

INGREDIENTS

Stir-fry

2 teaspoons	NONAROMATIC OLIVE OIL
1 Tablespoon	CHOPPED GARLIC
	FINELY CHOPPED GINGER
1 Tablespoon	FINELY CHOPPED LEMON GRASS
12 ounces	BONELESS, SKINLESS CHICKEN BREAST
1/4 + 1/8 tsp.	SALT
1/2 teaspoon	FRESHLY GROUND BLACK PEPPER
1/2	NAPA CABBAGE
1 cup	SMALL WHITE MUSHROOMS
1	RED BELL PEPPER

Sauce

1 cup	COCONUT CREAM (pp. 109–110)
1 Tablespoon	THAI FISH SAUCE OR LIGHT SOY SAUCE (see Buying, p. 32, n. 21)
1/2 cup	LOW-SODIUM CHICKEN STOCK (p. 225)
1 teaspoon	CORNSTARCH
1/8 teaspoon	CAYENNE PEPPER

BEFORE YOU COOK:

Finely chop ginger, garlic, and lemon grass. Wash chicken; dry on paper towel cut 2 inches x 1 inch. Wash cabbage, trim, and slice into 1/4-inch strips. Cut mushrooms in quarters. Cut red pepper in thin strips like matchsticks. Measure remaining ingredients.

COOKING METHOD

1. Heat 1 teaspoon of the oil in a large high-sided skillet on medium high. Add the ginger, garlic, and lemon grass, stirring to release flavors. Toss in the chicken, sprinkle with 1/4 tea-

spoon of the salt and pepper, and cook until white on the outside, about 2 minutes. Tip into a warm bowl, cover, and set aside.

2. Heat the remaining 1 teaspoon oil and stir-fry the cabbage, mushrooms, and red bell peppers until wilted but still crisp, about 2 minutes. Sprinkle with the remaining salt and pepper and add the chicken.

3. Combine the sauce ingredients and pour over the stir-fry, stir to mix, and heat to thicken. Serve with rice.

NUTRITIONAL ANALYSIS

Per serving: 238 calories, 24 g protein, 20 g carbohydrate, 7 g fat, 3 g saturated fat, 11% calories from saturated fat, 697 mg sodium, 5 g dietary fiber

AT A GLANCE
(FOR SKILLED COOKS IN A HURRY)

Heat large skillet. Add oil. Add ginger, garlic, and lemon grass. Sauté 2 minutes. Add chicken, season with salt/pepper, fry 2 minutes until white outside—set aside and cover. Add oil to pan. Stir-fry cabbage, mushrooms, and red pepper 2 minutes. Season. Add chicken. Combine sauce ingredients. Pour onto chicken. Stir to thicken for 1 minute. Serve over steamed rice.

Braised Chicken with Pasta

I first created this dish for rabbit, which now appears to be almost extinct (in the supermarkets). You can special order, but when I used chicken thighs in lieu, it was very good. By all means, you choose; either way, it's great with pasta. See notes on how to manage the calories.

INGREDIENTS

1 teaspoon	NONAROMATIC OLIVE OIL
1 (3-lb.)	RABBIT, cut in 8 pieces, or 3/4-pound boneless, skinless chicken thighs
3 ounces	CANADIAN BACON
1	ONION, finely chopped
2 cloves	GARLIC
2	RIBS CELERY
3	CARROTS, peeled
1	FENNEL BULB
1	RED BELL PEPPER
1/2 cup	PITTED, CHOPPED GREEK OLIVES (black)
1 (14 1/2 oz. can)	DICED TOMATOES IN JUICE
2/3 c. + 2 Tbsp.	NONALCOHOLIC WHITE WINE
12	FRESH SAGE LEAVES, chopped, or 2 teaspoons dried sage
2	BAY LEAVES
1/2 teaspoon	SALT
1 Tablespoon	ARROWROOT
2 Tablespoons	CHOPPED FENNEL FRONDS
2 Tablespoons	GRATED PARMESAN CHEESE
12 ounces	DRIED FETTUCCINE PASTA*

BEFORE YOU COOK:

Chop the Canadian bacon, onion, celery, carrots, and fennel into even-sized pieces. Crush the garlic. Measure remaining ingredients. Cook the fettuccine according to package instructions.

COOKING METHOD

1. Heat 1/2 teaspoon of the oil in a chef's pan on medium high. Brown the rabbit or chicken pieces on both sides, turning regularly. When golden brown, 5 to 10 minutes, remove to a plate.

2. Pour the remaining oil into the unwashed pan, add the bacon, and cook 1 minute. Add the onions, cook another minute, then add the garlic, celery, carrots, fennel, and bell pepper. Cook, stirring, 3 minutes. Stir in the olives, tomatoes, 2/3 cup of the wine, sage, bay, and salt, and bring to a boil.

3. Lay the rabbit or chicken pieces on top of the vegetables, cover, and simmer 45 minutes. Remove the meat to a plate to cool slightly. Pull the meat off the bones, shredding it as you go. Combine the remaining wine with the arrowroot and stir into the vegetable sauce. Heat to thicken, add the meat, and serve over pasta. Garnish with the chopped fennel and Parmesan cheese.

NUTRITIONAL ANALYSIS

Per serving: 541 calories, 60 g carbohydrate, 14 g fat, 3 g saturated fat, 5% calories from saturated fat, 706 mg sodium, 6 g dietary fiber

To cut carbs: Reduce by two carrots and reduce pasta to 1 ounce raw weight per serving. The pasta therefore becomes a garnish.

AT A GLANCE
(FOR SKILLED COOKS IN A HURRY)

Heat oil. Brown the chicken/rabbit meat (5–6 mins.). Remove to plate. Add oil; sauté bacon and onions. After 1–2 minutes add garlic, celery, carrots, fennel, and peppers. Stir 3 minutes. Add olives, tomatoes, 2/3 cup of wine, herbs, and seasonings. Boil. Lay meat on vegetable base. Cover and simmer 45 minutes. Pull meat off bones and shred. Add wine and slurry to vegetable dish with meat, and thicken. Use as a sauce over the pasta.

Chicken and Fennel Pie   SERVES 8

The "Maratimes" cover an area in the extreme northeast of Canada that borders the Atlantic Ocean. Call the area **pristine,** and you'd get it right. Community is strong, and home cooks still excel in good comfort foods like this original Rabbit and Fennel Pie. I converted it to chicken, but, please, if your supermarket will special order it for you, try the rabbit. Both meats are a wonderful combination of flavors with the fennel and mushrooms.

INGREDIENTS

Filling

2	FENNEL BULBS
1 Tablespoon	LEMON JUICE
1/2 pound	MEDIUM MUSHROOMS
2 teaspoons	DRIED MUSHROOM POWDER (see p. 31, n. 13)
1 1/2 teaspoons	NONAROMATIC OLIVE OIL, divided
1/2 cup	FLOUR
1/4 teaspoon	SALT
1/4 teaspoon	PEPPER
8	CHICKEN THIGHS (boneless)
1	ONION
3 cloves	GARLIC
2	CARROTS (1 1/2 c.)
2	RIBS CELERY (generous cup)
2 Tablespoons	TOMATO PASTE
2 cups	NONALCOHOLIC RED WINE

In Cheesecloth

2 teaspoons	HERBS OF PROVENCE
1/4 teaspoon	SALT
1/4 teaspoon	PEPPER

Pie Crust

1 recipe	GRAHAM'S BASIC PIE CRUST (see p. 229)

Note: Whole wheat phyllo can be used to greatly reduce both fat and carbs (p. 34, n. 33).

BEFORE YOU COOK:

Trim fennel (bulb only needed) and slice thick (1/2 in. to 1 in.). Halve the mushrooms. Wash chicken and dry on paper towels. Cut onions 1/4-inch dice. Crush garlic. Cut carrots diagonally in 1/2-inch slices. Cut celery into 1/2-inch pieces. Measure the rest and prepare the crust.

COOKING METHOD

1. Steam the fennel slices for 10 minutes. Lay the slices of steamed fennel in the bottom of a greased 9 x 13-inch baking dish or large oval baker. Heat the oil in a skillet on medium high. Pour the lemon juice into the hot pan and add the mushrooms. Cook until browned and tender, stirring often. Stir in the mushroom powder and scatter over the fennel in the baking dish.

2. Reheat the pan on medium and add 1 teaspoon of the oil. Combine the flour, salt, and pepper in a bag. Shake the chicken pieces in the flour until covered and tap off excess. Brown on both sides in the hot pan. Remove to a plate and set aside.

3. Sauté the onions in the same pan for 2 minutes, then add the garlic, carrots, and celery and cook 2 or 3 minutes more. Pull the vegetables to the side and add the tomato paste. Cook, mixing with the vegetables until the tomato paste darkens and coats all the vegetables. Pour in the wine and season with the salt and herbs of province. Lay the browned chicken on top, cover, and simmer 30–40 minutes or until the chicken is tender.

4. Remove the chicken to a plate to cool a bit, and slice evenly. Heat oven to 425°F. Lay the chicken on top of the mushrooms in the baking dish. Pour the baking liquid and vegetables over the top. Roll out the crust to fit the pan. Pinch the crust around the edges and prick the center with a fork. Brush the top with a little whole or 2% milk. Bake 15 or 20 minutes or until golden. Cut into 8 pieces and serve. Steamed broccoli and carrots would make up a really attractive plate. *(Note: Please also see Phyllo on p. 34, n. 33, for a different way to handle the crust.)*

NUTRITIONAL ANALYSIS

Per serving: 355 calories, 32 g protein, 28 g carbohydrate, 13 g fat, 3 g saturated fat, 8% calories from saturated fat, 280 mg sodium, 2 g dietary fiber

AT A GLANCE
(FOR SKILLED COOKS IN A HURRY)

Make a pastry* (p. 229). Steam fennel for 10 minutes. Use 9 x 13 bake dish. Line base with fennel. Heat oil in skillet. Sauté mushrooms with lemon and mushroom powder. Tip over fennel. Season/flour chicken. Sauté to brown. Remove. Add oil, sauté onion, then add vegetables with tomato paste. Stir to brown. Add wine and herbs. Return chicken. Cover, simmer 30–40 minutes until tender. Heat oven to 425°F. Pick out the chicken and allow to cool, then slice thickly (2–3 pieces). Lay it on top of mushrooms. Cover with vegetables and "sauce." Cover with pie crust, crimped at edges. Brush with milk. Bake 15–20 minutes. Cut to 8 servings.

   The "new" whole wheat phyllo pastry can be used to reduce fat and carbs (p. 34, n. 33).

Coq au Vin

If there ever was a well-known classic, surely this must be the Julia Child of a very short list. As simple as it gets—chicken in a red wine sauce—but don't forget the baby onions, the bacon, and oh, those herbs! This is splendid eating. Our recipe this time originated in Montreal.

INGREDIENTS

1/2 teaspoon	OLIVE OIL
1	3 1/2 POUND FRYER CHICKEN
10 ounces	PEARL ONIONS
3 ounces	CANADIAN BACON
2	MEDIUM TURNIPS
12	MEDIUM MUSHROOMS
1 pound	TINY NEW POTATOES, whole with skin
1/2 teaspoon	DRIED THYME
1/4 teaspoon	SALT
1/4 teaspoon	PEPPER
3	BAY LEAVES
1 1/2 cups	CHICKEN STOCK, low-sodium canned or homemade (p. 225)
1 1/2 cups	NONALCOHOLIC RED WINE
2 Tablespoons	ARROWROOT mixed with
4 Tablespoons	WATER (slurry)
1 pound	SPINACH LEAVES
2 Tablespoons	CHOPPED FRESH PARSLEY

BEFORE YOU COOK:

Wash the chicken; dry on paper towels. Cut in half. Peel onions (or use frozen). Cut bacon in 1/2 inch pieces. Cut turnip 1 inch. Wash and stem spinach. Measure remaining ingredients.

COOKING METHOD

1. Preheat the oven to 350°F. Heat the oil in a 10 1/2-inch chef's pan on medium. Brown the chicken, skin side down, turning once, about 5 minutes (it will be a tight squeeze). Remove from the pan and set aside.
2. Place the onions, Canadian bacon, turnips, mushrooms, potatoes, and thyme in the pan and cook, stirring, 2 or 3 minutes. Add the salt, pepper, and bay leaves and pour in the stock and wine. Return the browned chicken to the pan, and transfer all to a covered casserole. Bake in preheated oven for 40 minutes.

3. Remove the chicken to a plate to cool slightly before removing the skin and bones. Leave the flesh in the largest pieces possible. Discard the skin, bones, and bay leaves. Carefully strain the liquid into a fat strainer (retain the vegetables), then pour back into the pan (through a sieve) without the fat. Bring to a boil and let it boil, uncovered, 10 minutes to reduce the liquid. The vegetables will be sauce-like.

4. Stir in the slurry and return the cooked chicken. Place a handful of raw spinach leaves into each of six bowls and ladle the stew over the top. Sprinkle parsley on each serving.

NUTRITIONAL ANALYSIS

Per serving: 316 calories, 32 g protein, 31 g carbohydrate, 7 g fat, 2 g saturated fat, 6% calories from saturated fat, 707 mg sodium, 9 g dietary fiber

AT A GLANCE
(FOR SKILLED COOKS IN A HURRY)

Preheat oven to 350°F. Heat oil in skillet. Brown the chicken halves and set aside. Add oil; sauté onion, bacon, turnips, mushrooms, potatoes, and thyme (2–3 mins.). Add seasoning, bay, stock, and wine. Transfer to casserole with chicken. Cover and bake 40 minutes. Discard chicken skin and bones, and cut meat into largish pieces for six. Strain liquids (keep vegetables) and de-fat. Boil, thicken, and add chicken. Serve over uncooked spinach leaves.

Chicken a la Keene

There are several stories about where (or how) this popular recipe came together, but all of them clearly indicate its birthplace in Manhattan, New York City. The original is as rich as the style of the roaring twenties and their location. I've added both colors and textures and the use of yogurt cheese. It is lighter and to some extent brighter, yet it retains some of the creamy promise you'd expect of the original.

INGREDIENTS

Chicken

1	WHOLE FRYING CHICKEN (3 1/2 lbs.)
8 cups	WATER OR TO COVER CHICKEN
2 teaspoons	HERBS OF PROVENCE (p. 30, n. 8)
3 cups	CHICKEN BROTH (from cooked chicken)
1/2 cup	WILD RICE
1/2 cup	LONG-GRAIN WHITE RICE
1/4 teaspoon	SALT
3 cups	SNOW PEAS or SUGAR SNAPS

Sauce

3 cups	CHICKEN BROTH (from cooked chicken)
1	LARGE RED BELL PEPPER
12	MEDIUM MUSHROOMS
1/8 teaspoon	GROUND NUTMEG
1/4 teaspoon	SALT
1/4 teaspoon	PEPPER
1/8 teaspoon	CAYENNE
3 Tablespoons	CORNSTARCH mixed with
6 Tablespoons	WATER (slurry)
1 cup	NONFAT YOGURT CHEESE (p. 38)
	CHOPPED PARSLEY
	CHOPPED FRESH TARRAGON (optional)

BEFORE YOU COOK:

Rinse chicken and dry with paper towels. Measure rice, and chop pepper and mushrooms. Measure remaining ingredients.

COOKING METHOD

1. Rinse the chicken and place in a large pan. Cover the chicken with water, and add the Herbs of Provence. Bring to a boil, then simmer 1 hour or until tender. Skim off foam as it rises. Place the chicken on a plate and strain the broth. Pour 3 cups of the de-fatted broth into a saucepan and 3 cups into a 10-inch chef's pan. Save leftover broth for other uses. When chicken cools, remove skin and bones. Pull the meat into bite-size pieces.
2. Bring broth in saucepan to a boil; add wild rice and salt. Cover and cook for 30 minutes. Add white rice and continue cooking 15 minutes or until tender.
3. Bring broth in chef's pan to a boil, and reduce to 2 cups, about 10 minutes. Add peppers, mushrooms, nutmeg, salt, pepper, and cayenne, and simmer 2 minutes. Add the chicken. Stir in the slurry, and boil 30 seconds to cook the cornstarch. Place the yogurt cheese in a bowl. Stir 1 cup of the thickened sauce into the yogurt, to temper; then stir yogurt into sauce. Pour into the chicken mixture.
4. Serve with a 1/2-cup mound of mixed rice and steamed snow peas or sugar snaps. Garnish with parsley or tarragon.

NUTRITIONAL ANALYSIS

Per serving: 379 calories, 46 g protein, 34 g carbohydrate, 6 g fat, 1 g saturated fat, 2% calories from saturated fat, 387 mg sodium, 128 mg calcium, 3 mg iron, 245 RE Vitamin A, 94 mg Vitamin C, 1 mg Vitamin E, 3 g dietary fiber,

AT A GLANCE
(FOR SKILLED COOKS IN A HURRY)

Boil the chicken with Herbs of Provence and salt about 1 hour—skim. Place chicken on a plate to cool. Strain broth. Put 3 cups to saucepan, 3 cups to skillet. Remove skin from chicken; bone. Carve for six. In saucepan, boil, add wild rice, cook 30 minutes, then add white rice. Cook 15 minutes, until tender. In skillet, reduce to 2 cups, add vegetables and seasonings. Simmer 2 minutes. Add chicken and thicken. Pour a *little* hot cooking liquid into the yogurt cheese to temper the yogurt (see p. 38), then pour tempered yogurt into main chicken mixture. Serve over rice with snow or snap peas.

Curried Chicken with Sweet Potatoes and Bananas

*Now this was a **real** adventure! We took a small plane ride out into the South Pacific from Fiji to Wakaya, a small island in the midst of nowhere! At a tiny resort, amid laid-back luxury, we ate this dish, and then flew back to "normal life." It seems in retrospect to have been another world—and at $800 a night, it probably is!*

INGREDIENTS

Mango Sauce

1/2 cup	MANGO CHUTNEY
1/4 teaspoon	GARAM MASALA (p. 217)
1/8 teaspoon	CAYENNE PEPPER (optional)
5	QUARTER-SIZE SLICES FRESH GINGERROOT
3 ounces	DATES (about 12)
1	MANGO

Chicken

3/4 teaspoon	GOOD MADRAS CURRY POWDER
3	BONELESS CHICKEN BREASTS, skin on, about 6 oz. ea.
2 teaspoons	LIGHT OLIVE OIL
2 heads	BOK CHOY
3	BANANAS
1/3 cup	FRESH LEMON JUICE
12 ounces	STEAMED SWEET POTATO
1 teaspoon	ARROWROOT
1/2 cup	LOW-SODIUM CHICKEN OR VEGETABLE STOCK (pp. 225, 222)
2 cloves	GARLIC
2 teaspoons	GOOD MADRAS CURRY POWDER
1/2 cup	YOGURT CHEESE (p. 38)
4	GREEN ONIONS
9 ounces	PINEAPPLE WEDGES
1	MANGO

BEFORE YOU COOK:

Cut leaves off bok choy and remove the heavy white stems. Steam greens for 1 minute. Cool. Cut bananas into 1-inch pieces. Coat with lemon juice, and steam with sweet potato. Peel and thinly slice the ginger. Pit the dates and chop. Peel mango and fine dice. Peel, halve, and cut steamed sweet potato into 1-inch cubes. Make yogurt cheese. Cut green onions into 1/2-inch pieces. Thinly slice pineapple and mango for garnish.

COOKING METHOD

1. Mix mango chutney with the chopped dates, diced fresh mango, and the sliced gingerroot. Set aside for garnish.
2. Rub 1/4 teaspoon curry powder into the skinless side of each chicken breast.
3. Warm oil in a large frying pan. Sauté chicken skin side down for 2 minutes. Turn and cook another 3 minutes. Turn twice more, cooking for a total of 9 minutes, or until cooked through. Remove from the pan, and set aside. Do not wash the pan.
4. Combine arrowroot with stock to make a slurry.
5. Reheat oil and chicken juices in the large frying pan. Add garlic and curry powder, and stir until heated through. Deglaze pan with arrowroot slurry, loosening the flavorful bits from the bottom.
6. Spoon yogurt cheese into a 2-cup glass measure. Add a little hot stock and mix to temper the yogurt. Whisk in the rest of stock to make a smooth creamy sauce.
7. Reheat the bananas and sweet potatoes in a skillet and combine curry sauce. Keep warm but do not boil.
8. Remove and discard skin from chicken, and cut each into 1-inch pieces. Gently stir chicken and onions into banana mixture over medium-high heat.
9. Arrange two or three bok choy leaves on each plate. Place a serving of curry on bok choy and garnish with fine-sliced pineapple and mango slices. Mango chutney goes on the side.

NUTRITIONAL ANALYSIS

Per serving: 382 calories, 66 g carbohydrate, 6 g fat, 1 g saturated fat, 2% calories from saturated fat, 125 mg sodium, 7 g dietary fiber

AT A GLANCE
(FOR SKILLED COOKS IN A HURRY)

Combine mango chutney with fresh mango, dates, and ginger. Set aside for garnish. Rub curry powder into chicken breasts. Warm oil in large skillet. Sauté back and forth 9 minutes until 150°F internal. Remove. Reheat oil. Add garlic and curry powder. Deglaze and thicken. Temper the yogurt (see p. 38). Reheat the sweet potatoes and banana. Dice chicken into 1-inch cubes. Add. Toss. Combine with sauce. Stir gently. Serve over steamed bok choy leaves and garnish with fine sliced pineapple and mango. Serve the "enhanced" mango chutney on the side.

Recipes

MEATS

Beef Round Rump Roast

We went looking for the smallest roast of beef that would still roast well, carve well, and eat well—both hot and cold. It needed to be both lean and relatively tender and full of flavor. We eventually found the 3–5 lb. Rump (also called Round and Round Rump). It was splendid!

INGREDIENTS

1 clove	GARLIC
3 1/2 pounds	BEEF ROUND RUMP ROAST
season	SALT
season	PEPPER
2 teaspoons	THYME (dried)
1 teaspoon	OLIVE OIL
2 cups	SWEET ONION, finely sliced
4	FLOUR TORTILLAS (5-in. diameter)
4 Tablespoons	CREAM STYLE HORSERADISH
1/2 cup	DRY RED WINE (I like Merlot.)
2 teaspoons	ARROWROOT or cornstarch

BEFORE YOU COOK:

Allow beef to reach room temperature. Finely slice the onion. Cut garlic into fine slivers. Measure remaining ingredients. Preheat the oven to 375°F.

COOKING METHOD

1. Tuck the garlic slivers under the fat of the roast. Season the outside of the roast thoroughly with salt, pepper, and thyme.
2. Pour the onions into a baking dish. Add the seasoned roast, fat side up. Drizzle olive oil over the onions.
3. Place in the preheated oven for 30 minutes per pound to reach medium or slightly pink at 145°F on a meat thermometer.
4. After an hour, remove the onions and keep them warm.
5. Spread each tortilla with horseradish, cover with roasted onions, and set on a baking sheet in the oven to keep warm. Turn the oven off.
6. Remove the roast. Add the wine to the dish and scrape up the brown bits on the bottom. Turn into a small saucepan, skim off the fat, and thicken with arrowroot or cornstarch moistened with water (see p. 37, n. 7).
7. Place an onion-topped tortilla on each of 4 plates. Carve the beef in thin slices and serve 2 slices on each tortilla. Pass the wine sauce separately.

NUTRITIONAL ANALYSIS

Per serving: 301 calories, 30 g protein, 12 g carbohydrates, 13 g fat, 5 g saturated fat, 304 mg sodium, 39 mg calcium, 3 mg iron, 13 RE Vitamin A, 2 mg Vitamin C, 1 mg Vitamin E, 1 g fiber

AT A GLANCE
(FOR SKILLED COOKS IN A HURRY)

Preheat oven 375°F. Season roast with salt, pepper, thyme. Slice garlic and onion, stud meat with garlic; surround roast with onion. Roast 30 minutes per pound to 145°F (internal) for pink. Remove onions. Spread tortillas with horseradish. Deglaze roast pan with wine; thicken arrowroot. Heat tortillas. Carve and serve 3 1/2 to 4-ounce portions.

London Broil in Wine and Mushroom Sauce

SERVES 4

There is a trap here: some markets have a habit of selling a slice of top round of beef and calling it London Broil, but it really isn't. The authentic London Broil is also called skirt steak and is always thick (1–1 1/2 in.) at one end and less than 1/4 inch at the other. The meat grain runs from top to bottom and when cooked must be cut (carved) on the diagonal to be enjoyed. It has great flavor and relative tenderness when properly cut and is much less expensive than other premium cuts.

INGREDIENTS

1 teaspoon	OLIVE OIL
1/2 pound	WHITE MUSHROOMS (1-in. caps)
spray	OLIVE OIL SPRAY
1 teaspoon	DRIED DILL WEED
1 teaspoon	FRESHLY SQUEEZED LEMON JUICE
Optional	
2 teaspoons	WILD MUSHROOM POWDER (see p. 31)
1 1/2 pounds	LONDON BROIL (also called skirt steak)
1 clove	GARLIC, crushed
1/2 cup	TOMATO KETCHUP
1 Tablespoon	PARSLEY STALKS
1/2 cup	DRY WHITE WINE (de-alcoholized—see p. 32, n. 19)

BEFORE YOU COOK:

Wash and dry mushrooms, and slice 1/4-inch thick. Rinse the beef and dry with paper towels. Measure remaining ingredients.

COOKING METHOD

1. Heat a large skillet on medium-high. Add oil and toss in the mushrooms. Sprinkle with dill, lemon, and mushroom powder if you are using it. Spray with a little extra oil. Cook 2 minutes *maximum.*
2. Remove the mushrooms. Reheat the pan on high, 300°F.
3. Spray the steak with oil and sear it on both sides, 2 minutes per side. Add garlic to the pan and cook 1 minute. Add ketchup and turn steak back and forth for 2 minutes. Pour in wine and parsley stalks, and continue turning for 2 more minutes.
4. Remove the steak—it should be at 140°F or just pink. Cook less for medium rare.
5. Add the pre-cooked mushrooms to the pan and reheat. Carve the steak diagonally and serve with the mushroom-wine sauce.

NUTRITIONAL ANALYSIS

Per serving: 339 calories, 39 g protein, 11 g carbohydrates, 14 g fat, 5 g saturated fat, 450 mg sodium, 20 mg calcium, 3 mg iron, 36 RE Vitamin A, 6 mg Vitamin C, 1 mg Vitamin E, 1 g fiber

AT A GLANCE
(FOR SKILLED COOKS IN A HURRY)

Heat large pan and add oil. Sauté mushrooms with dill, lemon, and wild mushroom powder. Remove. Spray steak; sear both sides. Add garlic to pan. Add ketchup and parsley stalks. Turn back and forth to glaze. Add wine and reduce. Remove steak and add mushrooms. Carve diagonally in thin slices (1/4-in.). Serve sauce on side.

Steak and Oyster Pie

I love meat pies. The trouble is, they don't love me! Yet I want-my-pie-and-eat-it-too, so I've worked on the crust to make it both simple to fix, flaky, tender, and low fat. It took quite a time. Then I had to accept the idea of the crusted top being baked separately and added to the "stewed center" as a decoration. It actually works for me—how about you?

INGREDIENTS

1/2 recipe	BASIC PIE CRUST* (p. 229)
1 (10-oz.) jar	MEDIUM OYSTERS
1 teaspoon	NONAROMATIC OLIVE OIL, divided
1 medium	ONION
4	CARROTS
1/2 pound	TURNIPS
3/4 pound	MEDIUM MUSHROOMS
3/4 pound	LEAN CHUCK STEAK (trimmed of all fat and cut in 1/2-in. chunks)
2 heaping tsps.	TOMATO PASTE
2 cups	LOW-SODIUM CANNED OR HOMEMADE BEEF STOCK (p. 226)
1/4 teaspoon	SALT
1/8 teaspoon	PEPPER
2 teaspoons	HERBS OF PROVENCE
2 Tablespoons	ARROWROOT mixed with
1/4 cup	BEEF BROTH OR WATER (slurry)

*Or use the new whole wheat phyllo pastry to cut fat and carbs (p. 34, n. 33).

BEFORE YOU COOK:

Make the pie crust (see p. 229). Cut oysters in half. Cut onions in 1-inch chunks. Cut carrots and turnips in 1/2-inch slices. Cut small mushrooms in half. Trim the beef of all edible fat and cut in 1/2-inch pieces. Measure remaining ingredients.

COOKING METHOD

1. Preheat the oven to 400°F. Make the whole pie crust recipe and freeze half for another use. Roll the crust into a 9-inch circle. Wrap it around your rolling pin and transfer to a baking sheet. Make a scalloped edge by pinching it all around with your fingers. Cut into 8 equal wedges (leaving it in the round shape) and bake 10 minutes or until light gold and crisp. Set aside. Drain and chop the oysters, reserving the juice.

2. Heat 1/2 teaspoon of the oil in a high-sided skillet on medium high. Sauté the onions briskly to color for 2 to 3 minutes. Add the carrots, turnips, and mushrooms and sauté 1 more minute. Turn out onto a plate.
3. Heat the remaining oil in the same skillet on high. Toss in the meat and brown on 1 side 3 minutes. When it's nice and brown, stir in the tomato paste and cook until the paste darkens, 8 minutes. Add the vegetables to the meat and pour in the stock, oyster liquid, salt, herbs, and pepper. Cover and simmer 1 1/2 hours or until the meat is tender.
4. Stir in the slurry to thicken the mixture. Add the chopped oysters. Turn into a 9-inch round serving dish. Lay the cooked crust wedges on top and bake 6 minutes more before serving.

NUTRITIONAL ANALYSIS

Per serving: 276 calories, 21 g protein, 21 g carbohydrate, 12 g fat, 3 g saturated fat, 8% calories from saturated fat, 257 mg sodium, 2 g dietary fiber

AT A GLANCE
(FOR SKILLED COOKS IN A HURRY)

Make pastry (p. 229). Roll out to 9-inch circle and place on bake sheet. Crimp the outer rim. Cut into 8 wedges. Bake 400°F for 10 minutes. Cool on a rack.

Heat oil. Sauté onion. Add carrots, turnips, mushrooms and sauté. Turn out.

Add oil and heat high (300°F plus). Add meat and brown on 1 side. Add tomato paste and brown. Return vegetables and season. Cover and simmer 1 1/2 hours. Stir in slurry. Add oysters. Turn into 9-inch serving dish and top with crust. Bake 5 minutes. Serve.

North African Beef Bake and Matzo Dumplings

SERVES 4

We were served this dish during our first visit to Israel. We enjoyed such wonderful hospitality, and the market in Jerusalem was a real treat. No wonder we are called to pray for Jerusalem. Should peace come, it would be the world's number one destination for many reasons. The shank meat provides the smooth texture, the combination of kidney beans and barley is unusual, and you've got to try the matzo dumplings!

INGREDIENTS

1 teaspoon	NONAROMATIC OLIVE OIL
12 ounces	BEEF SHANK MEAT
1/4 teaspoon	FRESHLY GROUND BLACK PEPPER
1	ONION, roughly chopped
2 cloves	GARLIC
2	LARGE CARROTS
1/2 cup	DRY RED KIDNEY BEANS*
1/2 cup	BARLEY
2	TURKISH BAY LEAVES
6 cups	WATER
1/2 teaspoon	SALT
1 cup	FROZEN PEAS
	MATZO DUMPLINGS (p. 183)

Dried sour cherries can be used for variety as an alternative.

BEFORE YOU COOK:

Cut shank meat in 8 large pieces. Crush garlic. Cut carrots into 1-inch pieces. Soak beans overnight or use canned (if you must!). Rinse the barley. Make up the matzo dumplings (p. 183).

COOKING METHOD

1. Preheat the oven to 350°F. Heat 1/2 teaspoon of the oil in a high-sided skillet on high. Drop the meat in to brown on one side, about 3 minutes. Remove the meat to a plate and set aside. Reduce the heat to medium high, add the remaining 1/2 teaspoon of the oil to the pan and toss in the onions. Sauté, turning often. After 2 or 3 minutes, add the garlic and cook 1 minute more.

2. Return the meat to the pan. Add the carrots, kidney beans, barley, bay leaves, water, and salt. Bring to a boil, skimming off any foam that rises as it heats. Turn into a roast pan, cover, and cook in the preheated oven for 1 hour.

3. When the stew has cooked for an hour, add matzo dumplings. Spoon the stew over the top and return the pan, uncovered, to the oven for 1 more hour.
4. Stir in the peas and serve.

NUTRITIONAL ANALYSIS

Per serving: 377 calories, 26 g protein, 57 g carbohydrate, 5 g fat, 1 g saturated fat, 3% calories from saturated fat, 611 mg sodium, 12 g dietary fiber

AT A GLANCE
(FOR SKILLED COOKS IN A HURRY)

Preheat oven to 350°F. Heat oil. Sauté beef to brown. Remove to plate. Add remaining oil and sauté onion and garlic. Return meat. Add carrot, kidney beans, barley, bay leaves, water, and salt. Boil; skim. Turn into a roast pan and bake 1 hour. Add dumplings. Spoon juices over them. Return to oven for second hour. Stir in thawed peas and serve.

Matzo Dumplings
SERVES 4

INGREDIENTS

1/2 cup	MATZO MEAL
1/4 teaspoon	SALT
1/2 teaspoon	BAKING POWDER
1/2 cup	EGG SUBSTITUTE
1 teaspoon	NONAROMATIC OLIVE OIL

COOKING METHOD

Combine the matzo meal, salt, baking powder, egg substitute, and oil. Refrigerate 30 minutes. Form 8 dumplings using 2 dessert spoons and drop into a pan of boiling soup or stew. Reduce the heat to medium and boil gently for 15 minutes.

NUTRITIONAL ANALYSIS

Per serving: 90 calories, 1 g fat, 0 g saturated fat, 1% calories from saturated fat, 15 g carbohydrates, 1 g fiber, 256 mg sodium

Blade Steak and Beer Stew

We discovered this recipe in Northern Thailand, where its robust seasonings are pretty normal. When we applied it to our local beef, it made the typical-looking beef stew into a meal to remember and keep on repeating. It's become a favorite flavor.

INGREDIENTS

1 pound	STEW MEAT FROM A BLADE ROAST, cut in 1-inch cubes
1/2 teaspoon	NONAROMATIC OLIVE OIL
1 inch	GINGERROOT
1	ONION, chopped
2 cloves	GARLIC
1 Tablespoon	FINELY GRATED LEMON ZEST
4 teaspoon	TOMATO PASTE
1 (12-oz. can)	NONALCOHOLIC BEER (amber if possible)
1/8 teaspoon	GROUND CINNAMON
1/4 teaspoon	FRESHLY GROUND BLACK PEPPER
2	BAY LEAVES
4	MEDIUM CARROTS, peeled and cut
2	MEDIUM TURNIPS, peeled and cut in 1-inch chunks
1 Tablespoon	THAI FISH SAUCE (nam pla)
1 teaspoon	ARROWROOT MIXED WITH 1 TABLESPOON WATER (slurry)
1 teaspoon ea.	CHOPPED FRESH PARSLEY, CILANTRO, SPEARMINT and RED PEPPER FLAKES (optional), mixed

BEFORE YOU COOK:

Trim all visible fat from the beef and cut 1-inch cubes. Peel ginger, slice thinly. Crush garlic, chop onion, cut carrots and turnips in 1-inch chunks. Chop the fresh herbs.

COOKING METHOD

1. Heat 1 tablespoon of the oil in a high-sided skillet on medium high. Just as it starts to smoke, drop in the chunks of stew meat and allow to brown on one side only without stirring. The meat is ready when it is nice and brown on one side and has started to lighten in color around the edges, around 3 minutes. Remove the meat to a plate and set aside.
2. Add the remaining 1/2 teaspoon oil to the pan without cleaning it out, and reduce the heat to medium. Stir-fry the ginger, onion, garlic, and lemon zest together for about a minute. Add

the tomato paste, stirring until it darkens. Return the meat and any accumulated juices to the pan and pour in the beer. Stir in the cinnamon, pepper, and bay leaves. Cover and simmer for 1 hour and 30 minutes or until the meat is tender.

3. Add the vegetables and fish sauce, cover, and continue cooking for 30 minutes or until the vegetables are soft.

4. Stir in the slurry, allow to thicken, and serve over rice. Dust each serving liberally with the minced fresh herbs. For those who can't resist spicy heat, a sprinkle of crushed red peppers will do nicely.

NUTRITIONAL ANALYSIS

Per serving: 244 calories, 13 g carbohydrate, 7 g fat, 2 g saturated fat, 7% calories from saturated fat, 485 mg sodium, 3 g dietary fiber

AT A GLANCE
(FOR SKILLED COOKS IN A HURRY)

Brown beef on one side; remove. Add oil. Stir-fry ginger, onion, garlic, and lemon zest for 1–2 minutes. Add tomato paste; brown. Return meat plus juices to pan with beer. Add cinnamon, pepper, and bay. Cover and simmer for 1 hour 30 minutes until tender. Add vegetables and fish sauce; cook 30 minutes. Thicken and serve over rice. Dust well with herbs.

Vegetable Stew with Beef

This is another red meat recipe just to prove that treats are possible when the portion size is both reasonable and accompanied by a rich variety of vegetables. The liquid used is a nonalcoholic dry red wine, which adds to the balanced approach—and its great taste!

INGREDIENTS

2 Tablespoons	OLIVE OIL, divided
1 1/2 medium	YELLOW ONIONS
2	GARLIC CLOVES, crushed
3 cups	CARROTS
3 cups	RUTABAGA
1 Tablespoon	HERBS OF PROVENCE
2 teaspoons	SALT
2 1/2 pounds	BEEF CHUCK ROAST (or blade steak)
5 Tablespoons	TOMATO PASTE
2 cups	DRY RED NONALCOHOLIC WINE
1 Tablespoon	CORNSTARCH (or arrowroot, mixed to "cream" with a little water)

BEFORE YOU COOK:

Rinse the beef and dry with paper towels. Trim off all visible fat, about 11 ounces. Remove bone, 5 oz., and keep for stocks. Cut remaining lean meat into 1 to 1 1/2-inch cubes. Peel all vegetables (save trim for stock) and cut into even-sized cubes (1-in.). Measure remaining ingredients.

COOKING METHOD

1. Heat a large skillet to 300°F. Add 1 tablespoon of the oil to heat.
2. Add onion to sauté until brown, 10 minutes. Stir in garlic. Stir in the carrot, rutabaga, herbs, and salt.
3. Turn the vegetables into a bowl. Add 2 teaspoons of the oil and heat to 350°F smoke point. Add beef cubes one at a time, keeping space between them. Brown thoroughly *on one side.* Remove and repeat until all the beef is well browned. Remove the last batch.
4. Add the remaining teaspoon of oil to the hot skillet. Add tomato paste to oil and stir to darken for about 5 minutes (see p. 33, n. 27). Pour the red wine into the tomato paste to dissolve. Return the beef and vegetables, stir well, cover, and simmer (200°F) for 2 hours.
5. When the meat and vegetables are tender, bring to a boil and stir in the cornstarch "cream." Stir for 30 seconds to clear and thicken the sauce. Spoon 3 pieces of meat and 3/4 cup of vegetables into each bowl. Top with sauce.

NUTRITIONAL ANALYSIS

Per serving: 360 calories, 25 g protein, 12 g carbohydrates, 23 g fat, 9 g saturated fat, 550 mg sodium, 51 mg calcium, 3 mg iron, 994 RE Vitamin A, 17 mg Vitamin C, 2 mg Vitamin E, 3 g fiber

AT A GLANCE
(FOR SKILLED COOKS IN A HURRY)

Trim fat. Cut lean meat into 1–1 1/2-inch cubes. Sauté onion 10 minutes. Add garlic. Add carrot, rutabaga, herbs, and salt. Turn out. Oil pan to sear beef on one side. Turn out. Fry tomato paste to deep color. Add wine to dissolve paste. Return meat and vegetables, stir, cover, and simmer 2 hours. Thicken and serve.

Boiled Brisket of Beef and Cabbage

This is about as British as you can get. Our turn to retest this dish came as the temperature plunged to 20°F. What a welcome dish it made!

INGREDIENTS

2 Tablespoons	HERBS OF PROVENCE
2 1/2–3 lbs	BRISKET OF BEEF
2 cups	TURNIPS

(Note: Vegetables for 2 because you might want to have one hot dinner and save the rest of the meat for sandwiches.) Just multiply vegetables for a crowd.

2 cups	RUTABAGA
2 cups	CARROT
4 cups (estimated)	CABBAGE
1 Tablespoon	PARSLEY
season	PREPARED MUSTARD (Colemans)

BEFORE YOU COOK:

If the brisket is vacuum packed in a brine solution, take straight from the package and add to boiling "herbed" water (see cooking method section). Peel and cut hard vegetables into 1- to 2-inch chunks. Cut cabbage into 2 large wedges.

COOKING METHOD

1. In a large saucepan, bring enough water to cover meat by at least 2 inches to a boil with the herbs. Add the beef, reboil, cover, and reduce to a simmer (about 200°F) for 25 minutes per pound until internal temperature reaches 170°F.
2. Add the vegetables 30 minutes before cooking ends. If you don't have enough space, wait until the meat is cooked, remove it to a plate, and add the vegetables to the cooking liquid to boil for about 30 minutes or until tender.
3. Slice the brisket in 1/4-inch slices (2 slices usually make a 3-oz. serving). Surround the meat with the vegetables, dust with parsley, and serve an English mustard on the side.

NUTRITIONAL ANALYSIS   FOR FRESH BRISKET

Per serving: 202 calories, 28 g protein, 9 g carbohydrates, 6 g fat, 2 g saturated fat, 94 mg sodium, 53 mg calcium, 3 mg iron, 833 RE Vitamin A, 29 mg Vitamin C, 0 mg Vitamin E, 3 g fiber

NUTRITIONAL ANALYSIS FOR CORNED BRISKET

Per serving: 253 calories, 17 g protein, 9 g carbohydrates, 16 g fat, 5 g saturated fat, 1010 mg sodium, 55 mg calcium, 2 mg iron, 833 RE Vitamin A, 29 mg Vitamin C, 1 mg Vitamin E, 3 g fiber

AT A GLANCE
(FOR SKILLED COOKS IN A HURRY)

Combine herbs and water. Boil. Add brisket. Reboil, cover, and simmer for 1 1/2 to 2 hours (25 mins. per pound—internal temperature 170°F). Add roots and cabbage 30 minutes before end of meat cookery or cook after meat removed. Carve; surround with vegetable; dust with parsley. Serve with hot English mustard.

Bubble and Squeak
(cabbage, onions, potato, and corned beef)

SERVES 2

This dish remains firmly in the dark recesses of my life as a child during World War II in England. It's one way to use any beef brisket after its initial boiling (and after its use for sandwiches). Be sure to run the kitchen exhaust fan as it cooks—its aroma is powerful—but obviously I enjoy it (the taste that is)!

INGREDIENTS

1 Tablespoon	OLIVE OIL
1 cup	SWEET ONIONS
2	GARLIC CLOVE, crushed
3 cups	DRUMHEAD CABBAGE, finely sliced
2 cups	BOILED POTATOES
1/4 pound	COOKED CORNED BEEF
2 Tablespoons	PARSLEY
season	SALT
season	BLACK PEPPER

BEFORE YOU COOK:

Slice corned beef into 1/4-inch pieces and again into toothpick size. Finely slice the onion and the cabbage. Crush the garlic and slice the potatoes 1/4-inch thick. Measure remaining ingredients.

COOKING METHOD

1. Heat a large skillet, add oil, and heat on medium-high.
2. Fry onions for 4 to 5 minutes. Add garlic and cook 1 minute more.
3. Stir in cabbage and potatoes. Add brisket and push it down onto the skillet surface to brown.
4. Cover and cook together for 5 to 6 minutes to combine flavors. Add parsley, Worcestershire, and season to taste with salt and pepper.

NUTRITIONAL ANALYSIS

Per serving: 388 calories, 15 g protein, 43 g carbohydrates, 18 g fat, 5 g saturated fat, 1144 mg sodium, 119 mg calcium, 4 mg iron, 36 RE Vitamin A, 60 mg Vitamin C, 2 mg Vitamin E, 7 g fiber

Cottage Pie

This is just about as British as it gets—and everyone I know has their own little twist to the recipe. In order to keep the fats in their "proper" place, I subtracted 1/4 pound of minced beef and added 1/4 pound bulgur wheat, which has almost identical texture, and it really works—it almost sings!

INGREDIENTS

3 cups	CANNED OR HOMEMADE LOW-SODIUM BEEF STOCK
1/4 cup	BULGUR WHEAT
1 teaspoon	NONAROMATIC OLIVE OIL
12 ounces	EXTRA LEAN (9% fat content) GROUND BEEF
3 Tablespoons	TOMATO PASTE
1 1/2 cups	CHOPPED ONION
2 cloves	GARLIC
1 cup	FINELY CHOPPED CARROTS
1/4 cup	FINELY CHOPPED CELERY
1 teaspoon	DRIED THYME
1 Tablespoon	WORCESTERSHIRE SAUCE
1/4 teaspoon	SALT
4 teaspoons	ARROWROOT or cornstarch mixed with
2 Tablespoons	BEEF STOCK (slurry)
1 Tablespoon	CHOPPED FRESH PARSLEY
2 cups	MASHED POTATOES

BEFORE YOU COOK:

Finely chop all vegetables before you measure, then measure the lot! Make mashed potatoes.

COOKING METHOD

1. Preheat oven to 350°F. Heat beef stock and pour 2 cups over bulgur wheat. Set aside for at least 10 minutes to soften.
2. Heat a large skillet until very hot. Add 1/2 teaspoon oil, break the beef into small pieces, and add to the pan to brown. Mash the meat so it crumbles after it has browned. Reduce heat, stir in tomato paste, and cook until the paste turns dark red. Pour in the remaining cup of beef stock, and stir up flavorful bits from the bottom of the pan. Pour into a bowl.
3. Without washing the pan, heat remaining 1/2 teaspoon oil, and sauté onions. After 2 minutes, add garlic, carrots, celery, and thyme. Cook for 2 more minutes. Add Worcestershire sauce, bulgur with its stock, and cooked meat. Simmer 10 minutes, or until the carrots are tender. Stir in slurry to thicken. Tip into an ovenproof dish.

4. Cover filling with mashed potatoes, one spoonful at a time. Make designs on top with a fork. Bake for 20 minutes to heat through. Broil for 2 to 3 minutes to brown the top. Sprinkle with parsley and cut into 6 wedges. A classic side dish would be peas with mint and a broiled tomato.

NUTRITIONAL ANALYSIS

Per serving: 265 calories, 34 g carbohydrate, 7 g fat, 3 g saturated fat, 9% calories from saturated fat, 478 mg sodium, 5 g dietary fiber

AT A GLANCE
(FOR SKILLED COOKS IN A HURRY)

Preheat oven to 350°F. Heat 2 cups beef stock to boil. Pour over bulgur. Cover to soften off heat. Heat skillet very hot. Add oil. Add meat to brown. Reduce heat, add tomato paste, stir to darken. Add remaining stock. Turn out into bowl. Add oil, sauté onions, then garlic, carrots, celery, and thyme. Add Worcestershire, bulgur, and the meat. Simmer 10 minutes. Thicken. Tip into ovenproof "pie" dish. Cover (one spoon at a time) with mashed potatoes and mark top with a fork. Bake at 350°F for 20 minutes to heat. Broil the top to brown lightly.

South Central Chili

One could also call this Texas Chili since "South Central" really is all Texas (well, almost!). As a one-time Brit, I feel somewhat nervous about entering this bastion of regional individuality, but since the dish is made up of many hints from our new Texas family, we've taken the risk. The cocoa powder really works! Have fun, y'all!

INGREDIENTS

1 1/2 teaspoon	NONAROMATIC OLIVE OIL (divided)
8 ounces	BOTTOM ROUND
8 ounces	TURKEY THIGH
1	ONION, cut into 1/4-inch dice
1 (10 1/2-oz. can)	TOMATO PUREE
2	JALAPENO PEPPERS
1 (4-oz. can)	DICED GREEN CHILIES
1 teaspoon	GROUND CUMIN
1 teaspoon	DRIED OREGANO
1/4 teaspoon	CAYENNE PEPPER
1 Tablespoon	COCOA
1/4 teaspoon	SALT
1 1/2 cups	NONALCOHOLIC RED WINE (this can be replaced with beef stock)
1 1/2 cups	LOW-SODIUM BEEF STOCK (p. 226) OR WATER
3 cloves	GARLIC
1 Tablespoon	CORNMEAL
1 1/2 cups	COOKED BROWN RICE (p. 93)
3 cups	CANNED PINTO BEANS
Garnish	
1/2 cup	FINELY CHOPPED RAW SWEET ONIONS
1/2 cup	CHOPPED CILANTRO, garnish
6 Tablespoons	PARMESAN CHEESE, garnish

BEFORE YOU COOK:

Trim all visible fat from beef and turkey, and dice both 1/4 inch or finer (don't mince or process). Seed and fine-chop the jalapeno. Crush the garlic. Cook the rice (p. 93). Drain and rinse the beans. Finely chop the onion and cilantro. Measure remaining ingredients.

COOKING METHOD

1. Mix 1 teaspoon of the oil with the diced beef. Drop into a hot pan to brown. When it's well-browned, about 2 minutes, add the turkey and continue cooking 2 more minutes. Tip out onto a plate.
2. Heat the remaining oil in the unwashed pan and sauté the onion until it starts to wilt, about 2 to 3 minutes. Add the jalapenos, diced chilies, cumin, oregano, cayenne, cocoa, and salt. Cook 1 minute longer. Pour in the wine and stock, bring to a boil, reduce the heat, and simmer 30 minutes.
3. Stir in the garlic and cornmeal. Cook 3 or 4 minutes until the chili thickens. Divide the rice and beans among 6 hot bowls. Ladle the chili over the top and pass the garnishes at the table.

NUTRITIONAL ANALYSIS

Per serving: 377 calories, 48 g carbohydrate, 8 g fat, 3 g saturated fat, 5% calories from saturated fat, 877 mg sodium, 11 g dietary fiber. Carbs can be reduced by reducing the rice and beans by half.

AT A GLANCE
(FOR SKILLED COOKS IN A HURRY)

Mix 1 teaspoon oil with diced beef. Heat pan (300° plus). Sauté to brown. Add turkey and sauté 2 minutes. Remove to plate. Add oil and sauté onion. Add jalapeno, diced chilies, herbs, cocoa, and seasonings. Add wine and stock. Boil, reduce heat. Simmer uncovered for 30 minutes. Stir in raw garlic and cornmeal. Stir and cook 3–4 minutes to thicken. Ladle over rice and beans.

Roast Pork—Picnic Shoulder

*I chose this roast to see if its low cost per pound was still cheap when cooked, boned, and fat removed. It is! At just over $2.50 (U.S.) for cooked lean meat, it's a bargain. However, it's not easily carved and is probably best used for the **shredded** pork ingredient called for in many Mexican dishes. The crackling is a treat at one ounce–beyond that it threatens rapidly!*

INGREDIENTS

6 to 6 1/2 lbs.	PICNIC SHOULDER OF PORK (with rind)
1 teaspoon	HERBS OF PROVENCE
1 teaspoon	SALT
spray	OLIVE OIL (spray can)

Note: The cooked meat is best used as an ingredient in another recipe in quite small quantities 1 1/2 to 2 ounces (please see p. 34, n. 29).

BEFORE YOU COOK:

Wash the shoulder and dry on paper towels. Make parallel incisions through the rind about 1/4-inch apart and 1/4-inch deep with a sharp knife. Measure herbs and salt.

COOKING METHOD

1. Preheat the oven to 300°F. Sprinkle herbs and salt on outer skin. Spray with oil to just moisten. Brush or rub the seasonings into the incisions.
2. Set the meat on a rack over a baking pan and roast for 30 minutes per pound (about 3 1/2 hrs.) or until the internal temperature is 180°F.
3. Allow the roast to set for at least 15 minutes before carving. Cut away the crisp "crackling" from the top and scrape away and discard the surplus fat. (Serve the crackling only as a special treat–1 oz. crackling per person!)
4. Your 6-pound shoulder will contain 2 pounds of lean meat.

NUTRITIONAL ANALYSIS   3 OUNCES ROAST PORK

Per serving: 193 calories, 28 g protein, 0 g carbohydrates, 11 g fat, 4 g saturated fat, 68 mg sodium, 12 mg calcium, 1 mg iron, 2 RE Vitamin A, 0 mg Vitamin C, 0 mg Vitamin E, 0 g fiber

NUTRITIONAL ANALYSIS   1 OUNCE/28G CRACKLING

Per serving: 178 calories, 3 g protein, 0 g carbohydrates, 18 g fat, 7 g saturated fat, 10 mg sodium, 15 mg calcium, 0 mg iron, 1 RE Vitamin A, 0 mg Vitamin C, 0 mg Vitamin E, 0 g fiber

AT A GLANCE
(FOR SKILLED COOKS IN A HURRY)

Slash skin finely, brush in salt and herbs with a little oil. Roast 300°F for 30 minutes per pound until 180°F internal temperature. Set before carving. Best used in composite dishes.

Pork Tenderloin, South Island (NZ) Style

*I invented this dish way back when we lived in New Zealand during a time when venison was plentiful. Venison is now farmed and only **fairly** available, so I converted it to the pork tenderloin, one of the most versatile of all lean meats. The combination of blackberries with sage and thyme and a splash of balsamic "feels" like a game dish ought to be! (If you want to try it with venison, just chat it over with your meat market person; it may take a week to reach you.)*

INGREDIENTS

Blackberry Sauce

1 Tablespoon	HONEY
3/4 cup	FINELY SLICED SWEET ONION
1 Tablespoon	FRESHLY GRATED GINGERROOT
1/2 c. + 2 Tbsps.	ORANGE JUICE
2 1/2 cups	BLACKBERRIES (fresh or frozen)
1 Tablespoon	BALSAMIC VINEGAR
2	FRESH SAGE LEAVES
1 sprig	FRESH THYME (about 3 ins. long)
1 Tablespoon	ARROWROOT
1/2 cup	LOW-SODIUM BEEF OR VEGETABLE STOCK (pp. 226, 222)

Pork

1/4 teaspoon	SALT
1/2 teaspoon	FRESHLY GROUND BLACK PEPPER
1/2 teaspoon	SAGE
1/2 teaspoon	DRIED THYME
1 1/2 pound	TENDERLOIN OF PORK, cut into 12 medallions
1 teaspoon	LIGHT OLIVE OIL

BEFORE YOU COOK:

Finely slice sweet onions. Cut the pork into twelve slices and trim off any visible fat. Measure remaining ingredients.

COOKING METHOD

To prepare the sauce:

1. Bring the honey to a boil in a small saucepan over medium-high heat. When it is thick and bubbling, add the onion and ginger. Cook for a few minutes, stirring frequently, until the onions are soft and lightly browned.
2. As the sauce thickens, add 1/2 cup of the orange juice, slowly. Stir in the blackberries, balsamic vinegar, sage leaves, and thyme sprig. Simmer gently for 3 or 4 minutes, or until the berries are heated through and give up their juice.
3. Pour the sauce through a fine strainer set over a small saucepan. Press with the back of a spoon, discarding the seeds and pulp. You should have about 1 cup of juice.
4. Mix the arrowroot with the remaining 2 Tablespoons of orange juice to make a slurry. Add the slurry and the stock to the blackberry juice and set aside without heating while you cook the meat.

To prepare the pork:

1. Measure the salt, pepper, sage, and thyme into a large paper or plastic bag. Add the pork medallions and shake to coat.
2. Heat the oil in a large ovenproof frying pan. When the pan is very hot (300°F plus), brown the pork medallions for 2 minutes. Turn and brown the other side for 2 minutes.
3. Warm the sauce over medium heat, stirring frequently, until thickened and clear. Pour over the pork, stirring to capture the flavorful bits on the bottom of the frying pan.
4. To serve: Place two medallions of pork on each warmed dinner plate and spoon any extra sauce over the meat. Arrange portions of Mashed Sweet Potatoes (p. 104) and Spinach Defrosted in Broth (p. 102) on the side.

NUTRITIONAL ANALYSIS

Per serving: 361 calories, 30 g protein, 49 g carbohydrate, 5 g fat, 2 g saturated fat, 2% calories from saturated fat, 199 mg calcium, 4 mg iron, 2624 RE Vitamin A, 59 mg Vitamin C, 2 mg Vitamin E, 9 g dietary fiber

AT A GLANCE
(FOR SKILLED COOKS IN A HURRY)

Sauté the onion in very hot honey with ginger until soft. Add (slowly) orange juice, then blackberries, balsamic, sage, and thyme. Simmer 3–4 minutes. Sieve finely. Add slurry of orange juice and arrowroot to thicken and set aside. Bag season pork with salt, pepper, sage, and thyme. Sauté in hot pan 2 minutes, turn for another 2 minutes. Cover with sauce, stir well to deglaze pan, and serve.

Pork Tenderloin with Red Wine Sauce

Here we have a typical "down-home" southern Italian farmer's dish of pork, well-herbed tomato puree, a little wine, and polenta. I've used the cooked polenta that you can now buy made up in a roll like a short salami sausage. Just slice and heat. The convenience helps to make this combination a very simple evening meal.

INGREDIENTS

1 1/2 teaspoon	OLIVE OIL
1 pound	PORK TENDERLOIN
2	RED BELL PEPPERS
1/2 pound	MUSHROOMS
3 cloves	GARLIC
1/2 teaspoon	DRIED THYME
1/2 teaspoon	DRIED OREGANO
2	BAY LEAVES
6 Tablespoons	TOMATO PUREE
1/2 cup	NONALCOHOLIC RED WINE
4 slices	POLENTA (1-in. thick)
1 Tablespoon	ARROWROOT mixed with
2 Tablespoons	WATER (slurry)

BEFORE YOU COOK:

Trim all visible fat from the pork; keep whole. Chop the red peppers, quarter the mushrooms, and crush the garlic. Measure remaining ingredients.

COOKING METHOD

1. Preheat the oven to 350°F. Heat 1 teaspoon of the oil in a large high-sided skillet on medium high. Drop the tenderloin into the hot pan and brown on all sides, 4 minutes. Remove the meat to a plate and set aside.
2. Add remaining oil to pan, then add the peppers, mushrooms, and garlic to the same pan and cook for 2 minutes. Add the thyme, oregano, and bay leaves. Stir in the tomato puree and keep stirring while it darkens in color, 2 minutes. Pour in the wine.
3. Replace the meat in the pan and cover with sauce and vegetables. Lay the polenta slices around the pan and spoon vegetables and sauce over them. Cover and bake in the preheated oven for 30 minutes.

4. Remove the meat, slice on the diagonal, and divide among four hot plates. Set a polenta slice on each plate. Stir the slurry into the sauce and heat until thick and glossy, less than 30 seconds. Spoon over the meat and polenta. A good serving of just-steamed baby leaf spinach makes a great side dish.

NUTRITIONAL ANALYSIS

Per serving: 269 calories, 29 g protein, 20 g carbohydrate, 8 g fat, 2 g saturated fat, 6% calories from saturated fat, 247 mg sodium, 4 g dietary fiber

AT A GLANCE
(FOR SKILLED COOKS IN A HURRY)

Preheat oven to 350°F. Heat 1 teaspoon oil in large skillet. Brown tenderloin on all sides, turning often (4 mins.). Remove to plate. Add remaining oil, then peppers, mushrooms, and garlic to unwashed pan. Toss and cook 2 minutes. Add herbs, tomato puree, and cook to just darken. Add wine. Return meat, surround with polenta slices, and cover all with vegetable sauce. Cover and bake 30 minutes. When cooked, slice meat diagonally to serve 4. Thicken sauce; spoon over meat and heated polenta slice.

Pork and Shrimp Philippine Style

Treena and I have such fond memories of Manila, where we were the MCs at Lausanne II Conference. One evening we were invited to a private home to eat a decidedly local family-style dish. This is it—shrimp and pork with that curious underlying fish sauce flavor that we've come to celebrate and lots of peppers. I added the tofu just to see if it worked, and it did (unless you are terrified of tofu, of course).

INGREDIENTS

2 cups	WATER
3/4 pound	COOKED SHRIMP
1 teaspoon	PEELED AND CHOPPED GINGERROOT
1	RED BELL PEPPER
4	GREEN ONIONS
1/2 pound	PORK TENDERLOIN
1 teaspoon	NONAROMATIC OLIVE OIL
4 cloves	GARLIC
1/4 teaspoon	TURMERIC
2 teaspoons	FISH SAUCE
2 Tablespoons	ARROWROOT mixed with
1/4 cup	WATER (slurry)
3/4 pound	FIRM LIGHT TOFU
1/4 teaspoon	PEPPER
1 Tablespoon	CHOPPED CILANTRO
3/4 pound	THIN RICE NOODLES or angel hair pasta
as desired	RED PEPPER FLAKES (optional)

BEFORE YOU COOK:

Finely chop 1/4 pound of the shrimp. Peel ginger (reserve the peel). Chop the pepper (save the trim). Trim all visible fat from pork and cut into 1/4-inch cubes. Cut tofu to same size as pork. Crush garlic.

COOKING METHOD

1. Heat the water in a saucepan. Add finely chopped shrimp to the simmering water. Cut the ginger into thin strips and set aside, adding the ginger trim to the broth. Core, trim, and chop

the red pepper, tossing any trim into the simmering broth. Set aside the chopped pepper. Wash the onions and cut off and discard the root ends. Cut 3 inches off the green ends and add to the broth. Slice the rest and set aside. Simmer the broth for 15 minutes. Heat a large pot of water for the pasta while you make the sauce.

2. Heat the oil in a high-sided skillet on high. Add the pork, garlic, and ginger and cook for 3 minutes, or until the pork is lightly browned. Add the red pepper, turmeric, and fish sauce, and cook 1 minute longer. Strain the broth into the pan, add the slurry, and thicken. Stir in the tofu, the remaining shrimp, cilantro, green onions, and pepper.

3. Cook the noodles 3 minutes, drain, and divide among six bowls. Spoon the sauce over the noodles and serve with red pepper flakes on the side for those who like a little heat.

NUTRITIONAL ANALYSIS

Per serving: 346 calories, 55 g carbohydrate, 4 g fat, 1 g saturated fat, 2% calories from saturated fat, 439 mg sodium, 2 g dietary fiber

AT A GLANCE
(FOR SKILLED COOKS IN A HURRY)

Heat water in small pan. Add chopped shrimp with ginger, pepper, and onion trimmings. Simmer covered for 15 minutes. Heat oil. Add pork with ginger and garlic. Sauté 3 minutes to *just* color. Add peppers, turmeric, and fish sauce. Cook 1 minute. Strain broth into pork mix. Thicken. Add tofu (your choice), remaining shrimp, cilantro, green onions, and pepper. Serve over the cooked noodles.

Spicy Pork and Potato Casserole

Here is another "exotic" recipe from the Malay Peninsula in Southeast Asia. It's one of those adventures you can take if your family likes travel-eating (sitting at home and eating halfway around the world). The only odd ingredients are covered in the Buying section. If you like pork with a spicy twist, potatoes, and peanuts with a lime and coconut flavor, you'll love this recipe.

INGREDIENTS

1 1/2 teaspoon	OLIVE OIL
1 Tablespoon	SOUTHEAST ASIAN CHILI PASTE (see Buying, p. 34, n. 30)
3 cups	ONION
12 ounces	PORK TENDERLOIN
1 pound	RED POTATOES
2 teaspoons	GRATED LIME ZEST
6 inch piece	LEMON GRASS (See Buying, p. 34, n. 31)
1/2 teaspoon	COCONUT ESSENCE (see Buying, p. 33, n. 26)
1/4 teaspoon	SALT
2 cups	LOW-SODIUM CHICKEN STOCK
1 1/2 cups	YOUNG SOY BEANS (edamame) or frozen baby lima beans
2 cups	BROCCOLI FLOWERETTES
2 Tablespoons	LIGHTLY SALTED PEANUTS, chopped
1/2 cup	COCONUT CREAM (pp. 109–110)

BEFORE YOU COOK:

Trim pork of all visible fat and cut into 1-inch chunks. Cut small red-skin potatoes in half. Measure remaining ingredients. Bruise the lemon grass.

COOKING METHOD

1. Preheat the oven to 350°F.
2. Heat 1/2 teaspoon of the oil in a high-sided skillet on medium. Add the spice paste and cook for 1 minute. Stir in the onions and sauté until they soften and are covered with the spice paste, about 10 minutes. Bruise the lemon grass with the back of a knife to release the flavor and add to the onions with the lime zest and coconut essence. Remove to a bowl, scraping out all the onion but leaving any residue in the pan. Add the remaining 1 teaspoon oil, increase the heat to medium high, and brown the pork pieces on one side, 3 minutes.

3. Pour the stock into the pan with the pork and scrape up any brown bits on the bottom. Stir in the onion mix, potatoes, and salt. Cover and bake for 30 minutes. Uncover and continue to cook for 30 minutes or until the meat and potatoes are very tender. Discard the lemon grass. Stir in the broccoli and cook 6 minutes. Add the beans and heat through on top of the stove. If baby lima beans are used, add them with the broccoli. Stir in the coconut cream, scatter with peanuts, serve, and pass the spice paste for those, like Treena, who like it really hot!

NUTRITIONAL ANALYSIS

Per serving: 405 calories, 31 g protein, 45 g carbohydrate, 12 g fat, 3 g saturated fat, 5% calories from saturated fat, 8 g dietary fiber

AT A GLANCE
(FOR SKILLED COOKS IN A HURRY)

Heat oil. Sauté spice paste 1 minute. Add onion and sauté 10 minutes until soft. Add lemon grass, lime, and coconut essence. Remove to bowl. Add oil to unwashed pan on high heat and brown pork 1 side for 3 minutes. Add stock, onion mix, and potatoes. Cover and bake 30 minutes. Remove cover. Bake another 30 minutes. Add broccoli (6 mins.). Add beans to heat through. Stir in coconut cream; scatter peanuts. Serve spice paste on side for the "five-star" spice people!

Pork and Chicken Stew with Hominy, Mexican Style

Often called Posole, this is a much loved Mexican dish—almost a joyous celebration in itself and the result, some say, of a fabled accident. The "stew" itself is full of flavor, but when the herbs, hot peppers, limes, and raw onion are added, it's a real firework display.

INGREDIENTS

1 1/2 pound	PORK SPARERIBS
1/8 tsp. + 1/4 tsp.	SALT
1/8 teaspoon	PEPPER
3 1/2 pound	CHICKEN
1/2 teaspoon	LIGHT OLIVE OIL
1 cup	ONION
2 cloves	GARLIC
3	BAY LEAVES
1 29-ounce can	YELLOW HOMINY
1 bunch (8 c.)	FRESH KALE
Garnish	
1/2 cup	FRESH OREGANO LEAVES
3	LIMES HALVED
1/4 cup	DRIED CRUSHED RED PEPPER FLAKES
1/2 cup	FINELY DICED ONION
6	CORN TORTILLAS

BEFORE YOU COOK:

Rinse the pork and chicken; dry on paper towels. Roughly chop onion and crush garlic. Rinse and drain canned hominy. Wash kale; trim off heavy stalks; tear into small pieces.

COOKING METHOD

1. Preheat the oven to 350°F.
2. Season the ribs with 1/8 teaspoon of the salt and the pepper and place on a rack in a roasting pan. Add 1 cup of water to the pan, and roast in the preheated oven for 1 1/4 hours or until tender.

3. Warm the oil in a Dutch oven or large iron casserole over medium-high heat. Sauté the onions and garlic until the onion starts to soften, about 2 minutes. Lay the chicken on top of the onions and cover with 10 cups of hot water.

4. Add the bay leaves and the remaining 1/4 teaspoon of salt. Bring the liquid to a boil, reduce the heat, and cover the pot. Simmer for 1 hour. Turn off the heat, leave covered, and let sit for 20 minutes.

5. After the pork ribs have roasted, transfer them to a cutting board to cool. Add a little water to the roasting pan and deglaze with a flat-ended spurtel or wooden spoon, then pour the liquid into the pot with the chicken. Cut the meat off the ribs and roughly dice to 1/4-inch pieces or smaller.

6. Transfer the chicken to a large plate. Remove the skin and return it to the pot. Separate the legs and wings from the bird, and return the wings to the pot. Roughly chop the drumstick and thigh meat into pieces that can be easily eaten with a soup spoon. Remove the breast meat and cut into neat 1/2-inch cubes.

7. Return the carcass and any juices from the carving plate to the pot, along with the pork bones. Bring the stock to a vigorous boil for a few minutes to concentrate the flavors. Pour into a fat strainer a few cups at a time and allow the fat to rise to the surface. Pour the defatted stock (you should have 5 c.) into a large pot. Add the hominy, kale, pork, and chicken meat. Simmer for 5 minutes.

8. To serve, divide the posole among six warmed soup bowls. Pass small dishes of the fresh oregano leaves, lime halves, red pepper flakes, and diced onion for your guests to add according to their own tastes. Pass a basket of hot corn tortillas.

NUTRITIONAL ANALYSIS

Per serving: 444 calories, 38 g carbohydrate, 13 g fat, 4 g saturated fat, 7% calories from saturated fat, 540 mg sodium, 7 g dietary fiber

Note: The tortillas put the dish higher in carbohydrates but not over the top—your choice.

AT A GLANCE
(FOR SKILLED COOKS IN A HURRY)

Preheat oven to 350°F roast seasoned ribs for 75 minutes until tender. In larger saucepan heat oil and sauté onion and garlic. Lay chicken on top, cover with 10 cups of water, and add 1/4 teaspoon salt and bay leaves. Boil, cover, and simmer 60 minutes. Let cool in liquids. Strip meat from ribs and add pieced chicken (boil skin and bones in stock). Reduce the stock, strain, defat, and use 5 cups of reduced stock to heat hominy, kale, chicken, and pork. Simmer until kale is tender. Serve as a "soup" with the herbs, onion, lime, and hot peppers on the side.

"P3"—Pork Picnic Stewed with Pears and Red Peppers

I'm quite interested in this recipe because I obtained this meat from a partially trimmed pork picnic shoulder. The excess fat and skin were removed plus some of the meat. What I had was a large bone and 12 ounces of lean meat from a total 2 lbs. 11 oz. shoulder. But its cost per pound was only 99 cents. I had enough for four portions (3 oz.) and the blessing of the bone for stock. The meat is perfect for a stew because it contains lots of "melting" sinews that provide a superb texture and flavor for a simple stew.

INGREDIENTS

1 teaspoon	OLIVE OIL
2 cups	SWEET ONION, chopped
1 cup	CARROT, chopped
2 1/2–3 lbs	PART-TRIMMED BONE-IN PORK PICNIC SHOULDER (provides 12 oz. lean meat)
2 cups	CHICKEN STOCK
1	BOSC PEAR
1 large	SWEET RED BELL PEPPER
2 teaspoons	HERBS OF PROVENCE
1 teaspoon	SALT
1 Tablespoon	CORNSTARCH (or arrowroot)
1 c. tightly packed	BABY SPINACH LEAVES

BEFORE YOU COOK:

Cut pork meat from the bone; trim excess fat and discard. Cut meat into 12 to 15 1-inch pieces. Remove small bone for stock; retain big one for other uses. Chop the onion and carrot into large chunks. Cut the pear into 1/2-inch cubes. Finely slice the red pepper 1/4-inch or less. Measure remaining ingredients.

COOKING METHOD

1. Heat medium saucepan on medium high heat. Add oil to warm.
2. Toss in onions and carrots, and shallow fry for 10 minutes with the lid on.
3. Remove the vegetables and reheat the pan. Add pork pieces one at a time with spaces in between pieces to brown on at least one side.

4. Return vegetables to the meat and stir well. Add the small bone, chicken stock, herbs, and salt. Cover and bring to a boil. Skim off the foam and reduce the heat to a simmer (200°F–204°F). Cook for 1 hour.

5. Remove and discard the bone. Add the pear and peppers. Bring back to the slow boil, cover, and cook for 20 minutes. Stir in the cornstarch moistened with water (p. 37, n. 7) to thicken. Add spinach leaves and cook until wilted. Serve.

NUTRITIONAL ANALYSIS

Per serving: 211 calories, 19 g protein, 18 g carbohydrates, 7 g fat, 2 g saturated fat, 424 mg sodium, 41 mg calcium, 2 mg iron, 1059 RE Vitamin A, 81 mg Vitamin C, 1 mg Vitamin E, 4 g fiber

AT A GLANCE
(FOR SKILLED COOKS IN A HURRY)

Trim lean meat from large bone; cut away small bone. Heat pan and add oil. Sauté onion and carrot 10 minutes to brown. Remove. Sear meat well and return vegetables. Add small bone, stock, herbs, and salt. Cover and slow boil 1 hour. Remove bone. Add pear and peppers for extra 20 minutes. Add spinach. Stir in cornstarch to thicken. Boil 30 seconds to clear.

Pan Glazed Crosscut Baby Back Ribs (Pork)

SERVES 2–4

The barbecued baby back ribs are one of the most delicious (and messiest) of American down-home dishes. We set out to invent a simple indoor braised dish as either an appetizer for four or a supper for two. It works, even without firing up the grill.

INGREDIENTS

1 teaspoon	OLIVE OIL
1 1/2 pounds	CROSSCUT BABY BACK RIBS OF PORK
2	GARLIC CLOVES, crushed
1 Tablespoon	GINGERROOT, finely sliced
1/2 cup	TOMATO KETCHUP
1 cup	WHITE WINE (or de-alcoholized white wine)
1 Tablespoon	PARSLEY STALKS, chopped

BEFORE YOU COOK:

Rinse the pork and dry on paper towels. Crush the garlic; finely slice ginger (toothpick width). Chop the parsley *stalks* finely. Measure remaining ingredients.

COOKING METHOD

1. Warm the oil in a large skillet on medium-high heat.
2. Brown the ribs well on both sides, 10 minutes.
3. Remove the ribs and add garlic and ginger. Stir for 2 minutes.
4. Return the ribs to the pan and cover with ketchup. Turn back and forth to coat and brown slightly, 5 minutes.
5. Pour in the wine and stir to dissolve the tomato mixture. Cover and simmer 30 minutes.
6. Remove the lid, increase heat, and turn occasionally as the sauce reduces to a deep red glistening glaze. Dust with parsley stalks and serve with a fingerbowl if it isn't too culturally inappropriate.

NUTRITIONAL ANALYSIS – 2 SUPPER SERVINGS

Per serving: 664 calories, 75 g protein, 18 g carbohydrates, 26 g fat, 9 g saturated fat, 839 mg sodium, 54 mg calcium, 3 mg iron, 76 RE Vitamin A, 13 mg Vitamin C, 2 mg Vitamin E, 1 g fiber

NUTRITIONAL ANALYSIS — 4 APPETIZER SERVINGS

Per serving: 336 calories, 38 g protein, 9 g carbohydrates, 13 g fat, 4 g saturated fat, 420 mg sodium, 27 mg calcium, 2 mg iron, 38 RE Vitamin A, 7 mg Vitamin C, 1 mg Vitamin E, 0 g fiber

AT A GLANCE
(FOR SKILLED COOKS IN A HURRY)

Rinse ribs and dry. Heat skillet, add oil, brown ribs (10 mins.). Remove. Sauté garlic and ginger. Return ribs and add tomato ketchup. Turn to coat. Add wine and stir well. Cover. Reduce heat, simmer 30 minutes. Remove lid and increase heat. Reduce to a glaze and add parsley stalks.

Roast Half Leg of Lamb with Apple and Orange Sauce

*Having been raised in the U.K. with Welsh lamb and having lived in Australia, New Zealand, and near Ellensberg in Washington State, we are **obviously** fond of lamb. It's a firm family favorite. The sauce was created in New Zealand and named in honor of our son Andrew's birthday. We prefer to eat lamb at about 160°F internal temperature or barely pink.*

INGREDIENTS

3–4 pounds	LEG OF LAMB
1 teaspoon	FLOUR
1/2 teaspoon	SALT
1/4 teaspoon	PEPPER
1 teaspoon	HERBS OF PROVINCE
spray	OLIVE OIL SPRAY
1 large	GARLIC CLOVE
1 cup	UNSWEETENED APPLE JUICE
1 cup	100% ORANGE JUICE, unsweetened
1 Tablespoon	CORNSTARCH or Arrowroot

BEFORE YOU COOK:

Wash the lamb and dry with paper towels. Mix the flour with the seasonings. Peel and slice the garlic into 3 wedges.

COOKING METHOD

1. Preheat the oven to 350°F. Make sure the lamb is at room temperature. Slash the fat in an even diamond-shaped pattern 1 inch wide and 1/4 inch deep.
2. Combine the flour, salt, and pepper and dust lamb all over with the mixture. Spray with oil and brush it down into the cuts.
3. Make small incisions near the bone at either end and poke in the garlic wedges.
4. Put lamb in the oven and roast for 30 minutes per pound.
5. 30 minutes before the meat is done, pour the apple and orange juices over the meat.
6. When the internal temperature of the roast reaches 150°F, remove and let sit for 15 minutes. The temperature will rise to 160°F and the juices will set.
7. Pour the pan drippings into a fat strainer (p. 41, n. 6). Decant the juices into a small pan and discard the fat. Thicken lightly with the cornstarch or arrowroot mixed with a little cold water. Boil for 30 seconds.

NUTRITIONAL ANALYSIS

Per serving: 175 calories, 24 g protein, 7 g carbohydrates, 5 g fat, 2 g saturated fat, 195 mg sodium, 14 mg calcium, 2 mg iron, 14 RE Vitamin A, 14 mg Vitamin C, 0 mg Vitamin E, 0 g fiber

AT A GLANCE
(FOR SKILLED COOKS IN A HURRY)

Wash room temperature lamb, dry. Slash fat, dust with seasoned flour, and brush in seasonings with oil. Preheat oven to 350°F. Roast 30 minutes per pound to 150°F. 30 minutes before end, add orange/apple juices to coat. Make gravy (remove fat), thicken, and serve.

Moussaka

This is the famous Greek lamb and eggplant "pie." The crust is formed with an egg-based white sauce that, in modern times, has become larger and deeper and, as a result, fattier and richer! If carbs concern you, just replace the bulgur wheat with 1/4 pound of extra minced lamb. This is another whole meal in one.

INGREDIENTS

1 teaspoon	OLIVE OIL
1 cup	CHOPPED ONION
3 cloves	GARLIC
12 ounces	VERY LEAN GROUND LAMB
3 Tablespoons	TOMATO PASTE
1 teaspoon	DRIED OREGANO
1/4 cup	BULGUR WHEAT
2 cups	NONALCOHOLIC RED WINE
1/8 teaspoon	CINNAMON
1/8 teaspoon	SALT
1/4 teaspoon	FRESHLY GROUND PEPPER
12 ounces	EGGPLANT (peeled weight)
1/4 c. + 2 Tbsps.	GRATED PARMESAN

Topping

1 cup	1% MILK
2 Tablespoons	CORNSTARCH mixed with
4 Tablespoons	WATER (slurry)
1/8 teaspoon	NUTMEG
2 Tablespoons	EGG SUBSTITUTE

BEFORE YOU COOK:

Crush garlic. Mince the lean lamb. Peel and thinly slice (1/4 in.) the eggplant.

COOKING METHOD

1. Heat the oil in a high-sided skillet and sauté the onions for 3 minutes on medium high. Add the garlic and cook another minute. Remove the onions to a plate and reheat the pan.
2. When the pan is good and hot, crumble in the ground lamb and fry until brown. Add the tomato paste and stir until it starts to darken, 2 minutes.

3. Return the cooked onions to the pan with the lamb and stir in the oregano and bulgur wheat. Pour in the wine and season with the cinnamon, salt, and pepper. Bring to a boil and simmer 5 minutes.

4. Lay the eggplant slices on a bake sheet and sprinkle with 1/4 cup of the grated Parmesan cheese. Pan fry in a mist of sprayed oil, a few slices at a time on both sides to just brown. Set aside to cool.

5. Combine the milk, slurry, and nutmeg in a small saucepan. Bring to a boil and cook, stirring, until thick. Pull it off the heat and add the egg substitute.

6. Tip the meat mixture out of the pan into a bowl. Cover the bottom of a greased round cake tin with a layer of eggplant slices. Spread a cup of the meat sauce over the eggplant, sprinkle with a third of the Parmesan cheese. Make a second and third layer the same way with the meat sauce on the top. Make a shallow indentation in the top layer of meat sauce to hold the liquid topping.

7. Preheat oven to 350°F. Pour the custard sauce topping into the indentation without letting too much spill over. Sprinkle with the remaining Parmesan cheese and bake in the preheated oven for 25 minutes or until the topping is solid and the eggplant tender. Place under the broiler (or a very hot oven) for 5 minutes or until golden brown on top. Cut into 6 wedges and serve.

NUTRITIONAL ANALYSIS

Per serving: 239 calories, 17 g carbohydrate, 9 g fat, 4 g saturated fat, 15% calories from saturated fat, 211 mg sodium, 3 g dietary fiber

AT A GLANCE
(FOR SKILLED COOKS IN A HURRY)

Heat oil in skillet. Sauté onions. Add garlic; sauté. Remove to plate. Increase heat; add oil and lamb. Brown well. Add tomato paste and brown deeply. Return onions; add oregano and bulgur. Add wine, cinnamon, and seasonings. Boil, then simmer for 5 minutes. Coat sliced eggplant with cheese and oil pan with spray. Sauté to brown. Set aside. Combine milk, slurry, and nutmeg. Boil; stir to thicken. Cool a little. Add egg substitute and stir in well. Line 9-inch diameter greased cake tin with eggplant. Pour meat into base. Cover with sautéed eggplant and cheese, then meat in layers to meat on the top. Make shallow indentation to hold custard. Bake 350°F, 20 minutes to reheat. Increase heat to brown the custard.

Braised Lamb Shanks

All shanks produce extremely rich-textured meat. They owe their texture more to melted connective tissue than to fat. This is one of my all-time favorites. I usually slip it off the bone to serve it. One shank provides enough for the two of us, and with sweet potato and kale—ah! It's so good on a cold day.

INGREDIENTS

1 teaspoon	OLIVE OIL
2 cups	SWEET ONIONS
2 cups	CARROTS
2 cups	PARSNIPS
2 pounds	LAMB SHANKS
6 Tablespoons	TOMATO PASTE
3 cups	CHICKEN STOCK
2 teaspoons	HERBS OF PROVENCE
1 Tablespoon	CORNSTARCH
Optional	
1/2 cup	POM (pomegranate juice)

BEFORE YOU COOK:

Preheat the oven to 325°F. Wash shanks well and dry on paper towels. Cut the carrot, onion, and parsnips into about 1/2-inch pieces. Measure remaining ingredients.

COOKING METHOD

1. Heat a large skillet. Add the oil to warm.
2. Shallow-fry the onions, carrot, and parsnips for 10 minutes to color.
3. Remove from pan and build the heat to 300°F. Add the lamb shanks and brown on both sides, about 10 minutes.
4. Transfer the vegetables to an ovenproof casserole or dish. Place shanks on top.
5. Add tomato paste to the skillet without washing it. Cook until the color darkens, 5 to 8 minutes. Add chicken stock, stir out the lumps, and add the herbs. Pour over the shanks. Cover with foil.
6. Bake in the preheated oven for 2 hours. Turn once after an hour.
7. Remove the bones. Add the optional Pom or other red juice. Stir in cornstarch moistened with water (p. 37, n. 7). Serve with sweet potatoes and kale or a green leafy vegetable of your choice.

NUTRITIONAL ANALYSIS

Per serving: 385 calories, 24 g protein, 27 g carbohydrates, 20 g fat, 9 g saturated fat, 146 mg sodium, 60 mg calcium, 2 mg iron, 1662 RE Vitamin A, 29 mg Vitamin C, 3 mg Vitamin E, 5 g fiber

AT A GLANCE
(FOR SKILLED COOKS IN A HURRY)

Wash shanks and dry. Sauté onion, carrot, and parsnips 10 minutes. Remove. Sauté lamb shanks 10 minutes to brown. Put both in ovenproof dish. Brown tomato paste; add stock and herbs. Pour over shanks. Cover with foil. Bake 2 hours at 325°F. Slip off bone. Add cornstarch and Pom (or wine). Thicken. Serve green leaf vegetables and sweet potatoes.

Kheema: Minced Lamb Curry

*This is a great example of a simple recipe that **looks** complicated because it has 24 ingredients, but 14 of them are simply small amounts of herbs, spices, and seasonings. They are there to provide layers of flavor, not unlike the great perfumes provide layers of aroma. So **please** check out the At a Glance section before you judge a recipe by its contents!*

INGREDIENTS

2 teaspoons	NONAROMATIC OLIVE OIL
2 (3 c. chopped)	ONIONS
6 cloves	GARLIC
2 teaspoons	GRATED GINGER
1 teaspoon	GROUND CUMIN
1/4 teaspoon	GROUND RED PEPPER
1/4 teaspoon	TURMERIC
1 teaspoon	GROUND CORIANDER
1/2 teaspoon	SALT
12 ounces	LEAN LAMB
2 (1 c. sliced)	CARROTS
3	MEDIUM UNPEELED RED POTATOES
4 (2 c. chopped)	ROMA TOMATOES
1	SERRANO CHILE
2 Tablespoons	LEMON JUICE
1 cup	FROZEN PEAS, thawed
1 Tablespoon	ARROWROOT mixed with
2 Tablespoons	WATER (slurry)
1 teaspoon	GARAM MASALA (see next page)
1 Tablespoon	FRESH CILANTRO
1 Tablespoon	FRESH SPEARMINT

BEFORE YOU COOK:

Rough chop onion; crush garlic; grind the lean lamb (or process). Peel and thinly slice carrots. Cut potatoes into 1-inch dice. Core and chop tomatoes. Seed and finely chop Serrano. Chop herbs.

COOKING METHOD

1. Heat 1 teaspoon oil in a high-sided skillet. Sauté onions for 3 minutes, add garlic, ginger, cumin, red pepper, turmeric, coriander, and salt. Cook until onions are soft and golden, 5 minutes. Put in a bowl.
2. Without washing the pan, heat remaining oil. Crumble lamb into hot pan and brown on one side 3 minutes without stirring. Stir in carrots, potatoes, 1 1/2 cups tomatoes, chili, and sautéed onions. Cover and simmer 30 minutes.
3. Add lemon juice, peas, the remaining 1/2 cup of tomatoes, and 1 cup water. When boiling, stir in the slurry. Add garam masala to taste.
4. Garnish with the spearmint and cilantro.

Garam Masala

1/2 teaspoon whole allspice   1-inch cinnamon stick
1/2 teaspoon whole cloves   1/4 teaspoon ground nutmeg

Grind all ingredients together in a designated coffee grinder.

NUTRITIONAL ANALYSIS

Per serving: 504 calories, 66 g carbohydrate, 12 g fat, 3 g saturated fat, 4% calories from saturated fat, 477 mg sodium, 11 g dietary fiber. Carbs can be reduced by reducing the potatoes by half.

AT A GLANCE
(FOR SKILLED COOKS IN A HURRY)

Heat oil; sauté onion. Add garlic, five spices, and salt. Continue to sauté 5 minutes. In unwashed pan add oil and brown lamb on one side. Add carrot, potatoes, three-quarters the tomatoes, chili, and cooked onions. Cover and simmer 30 minutes. Add lemon juice, peas, remaining tomatoes, and 1 cup water. Thicken and add Garam Masala to taste.

A Mild Meat Curry (using shoulder of lamb)

*Treena is a passionate curry eater, and she **used** to like it very hot (spicy). I like it mild. We have now reached a democratic solution: it's made mild and jazzed with cayenne pepper later **if she must!** She is content with this recipe and so am I! Just replace the lamb with meat of your preference that comes from a "working" area (neck shoulder, shin, etc.).*

INGREDIENTS

2 teaspoons	OLIVE OIL, divided
1/2 pound	SWEET ONIONS
1 Tablespoon	FINELY SLICED GINGERROOT
2	GARLIC CLOVES, crushed
1 Tablespoon	MILD MADRAS CURRY POWDER
1 pound	LEAN LAMB SHOULDER
1 pound	BUTTERNUT SQUASH, peeled
1 teaspoon	SALT
2 cups	CHICKEN OR VEGETABLE STOCK
1/4 cup	RAISINS
1	BOSC PEAR
2 cups	EDAMAME BEANS (optional)
1 Tablespoon	CORNSTARCH
1 Tablespoon	PARSLEY

BEFORE YOU COOK:

Trim off all surplus fat and cut lamb into 1-inch pieces. Dice the onion and butternut squash. Crush garlic; slice ginger into toothpick-size pieces. Core pear but leave skin on, then dice 1/2 inch. Measure remaining ingredients.

COOKING METHOD

1. Heat a large skillet to 300°F. Add 1 teaspoon of the oil to warm.
2. Add onion. Shallow-fry for 5 minutes. Add ginger, garlic, and curry powder. Cook, stirring, for another 5 minutes to "warm" spices.
3. Remove onion mixture to a plate. Add the remaining oil. Increase the heat to high.

4. Sear the meat for 8 to 10 minutes or until it is quite brown. Replace the onion mixture and add squash and salt. Pour in stock and bring to a boil. Skim and cover to slow boil for 30 minutes.
5. Stir in the raisins, diced pear, and edamame, if you are using them. Cook, covered, for another 30 minutes.
6. Thicken with cornstarch (see p. 37, n. 7). Add parsley and serve.

NUTRITIONAL ANALYSIS WITHOUT EDAMAME

Per serving: 417 calories, 24 g protein, 39 g carbohydrates, 20 g fat, 9 g saturated fat, 666 mg sodium, 87 mg calcium, 3 mg iron, 554 RE Vitamin A, 16 mg Vitamin C, 1 mg Vitamin E, 5 g fiber

NUTRITIONAL ANALYSIS WITH EDAMAME

Per serving: 544 calories, 35 g protein, 54 g carbohydrates, 24 g fat, 8 g saturated fat, 673 mg sodium, 337 mg calcium, 7 mg iron, 577 RE Vitamin A, 54 mg Vitamin C, 1 mg Vitamin E, 10 g fiber

AT A GLANCE
(FOR SKILLED COOKS IN A HURRY)

Heat large skillet; add oil; sauté onion. Add garlic, ginger, and curry powder and warm spices 5 minutes. Remove. Reheat pan; oil and sear the meat 8–10 minutes to brown. Return onion. Add squash, stock, and salt. Boil, skim, reduce heat, cover, and cook 30 minutes. Add raisins, pear, and optional edamame. Slow boil 30 minutes. Thicken, taste, and add parsley for garnish. Serve.

Irish Stew, Shoulder of Lamb

The closer to the bone, the sweeter the meat! If that was ever a proven fact, it's with this neck and shoulder lamb recipe. Slow stewing buried in sweet onions, carrots, and barley produces one of the world's best "people" dishes.

INGREDIENTS

1 teaspoon	OLIVE OIL
1 large	SWEET ONION
14 ounces	CARROTS
1/2 cup	POT BARLEY
2 1/2 cups	CHICKEN OR VEGETABLE STOCK
1 pound	LEAN LAMB SHOULDER
2 teaspoons	SALT
garnish	CHOPPED PARSLEY

BEFORE YOU COOK:

Chop onion into 1/2-inch cubes. Cut carrots into even-sized 1 1/2 inch x 1/2 inch pieces. Dice lamb into 1-inch cubes. Wash the barley and drain. Measure remaining ingredients.

COOKING METHOD

1. Warm a medium-large saucepan on medium-high heat for 5 minutes. Add oil to warm.
2. Shallow-fry the onions until just brown, 5 to 8 minutes.
3. Add the carrots, barley, stock, and 1 teaspoon of the salt. Bring to a boil.
4. Add the meat (for a white stew, the meat isn't browned). Stir, cover, and bring to a boil again. Skim and reduce the heat to a low boil. Cook, covered, for 1 1/2 hours or until the meat and barley are tender.
5. Taste for seasoning (the barley soaks up the salt). Add parsley and serve. It's an all-in-one dish.

NUTRITIONAL ANALYSIS

Per serving: 352 calories, 21 g protein, 34 g carbohydrates, 15 g fat, 7 g saturated fat, 1276 mg sodium, 74 mg calcium, 3 mg iron, 2808 RE Vitamin A, 17 mg Vitamin C, 2 mg Vitamin E, 8 g fiber

AT A GLANCE
(FOR SKILLED COOKS IN A HURRY)

Warm saucepan; add oil and sauté onion. Add carrot, washed barley, and stock with salt. Boil. Add cubed lamb. Re-boil. Skim, cover, low boil for 1 1/2 hours. Adjust seasoning. Add parsley. Serve.

Recipes
STOCKS, ETC.

Basic Vegetable Stock

MAKES 1 QUART
(4 CUPS)

When I talk (often!) about nine servings of fruit and vegetables, I often get the response "But they are so expensive." While I may argue that "it depends what you compare it to," I will admit that when we peel hard vegetables, or discard outer leaves, we are throwing out real money. So why not use the peel and damaged leaves to produce a well-flavored stock for all manner of recipes? My vegetable stock is comprised of two techniques. The first is **collection;** the second, **concentration.**

Collection. Every time I peel a **washed** vegetable (the washing is vital!), I put the trim into a large plastic bag with other previously saved peelings and press down hard to exhaust the air and take up less space in the deep freeze. After 3 to 4 days, I have enough to make one batch, usually 2 quarts of stock.

Concentration. Having strained the vegetable trim, I'm now left with the two quarts of fairly lightly-flavored water. I then reduce it by boiling in an open saucepan to just one quart (4 c.). You can really taste the difference! I then use one of two different storage methods. The first is to decant 2 cups into a single zip-lock bag and date it. The second is to fill our old ice cube tray, freeze, and then turn out into a bag for use in tiny ways where needed.

Having two "kits" of both in our fridge is enough for general use. Any more trim is simply discarded or fed into the compost.

Now that we've dealt with waste, let's look at the very best basic vegetable stock you can make by **design.**

INGREDIENTS

1 teaspoon	OLIVE OIL	1/2 cup	CHOPPED CARROT
1/2 cup	CHOPPED ONION	1/2 cup	CHOPPED TURNIP
2 cloves	GARLIC, crushed	1/4 cup	CHOPPED LEEKS
1 root	GINGER, grated	3 sprigs	PARSLEY
1/2 cup	CHOPPED CELERY		SEASON TO TASTE

COOKING METHOD

1. Heat stockpot (enough for 8 c. water). Add oil, onion, and garlic, and sauté for 5 minutes.
2. Add the remaining ingredients. Boil and then simmer for 3 minutes, using 5 cups of *filtered* water.
3. Strain and use, or freeze for future use.

Note: This, I admit, is a "special" stock, with very little herbal influence—that will be up to you to select for that special dish. It is useful to compare the vegetable trim stock with this premium stock. Both are infinitely better than tap water!

Basic Fish or Shrimp Stock

INGREDIENTS

1 teaspoon	NONAROMATIC OLIVE OIL
1	ONION, peeled and chopped
1/2 cup	CELERY TOPS, coarsely chopped
2 sprigs	FRESH THYME or 1 teaspoon dried thyme
1	BAY LEAF
1 pound	FISH BONES (no heads) OR SHRIMP SHELLS
6	BLACK PEPPERCORNS
2	WHOLE CLOVES
5 cups	WATER

COOKING METHOD

1. Pour the oil into a large saucepan and sauté the onion, celery tops, thyme, and bay leaf until onion is translucent, about 5 minutes. To ensure a light-colored stock, be careful not to brown.
2. Add the fresh bones or shrimp shells, peppercorns, and cloves. Cover with 5 cups water, bring to a boil, reduce the heat, and simmer for 25 minutes.
3. Strain through a fine mesh sieve and cheesecloth.

NUTRITIONAL ANALYSIS

Per Serving: 13 calories, 1 g fat, 0 g saturated fat, 0% calories from saturated fat, 0 g carbohydrate, 0 g dietary fiber, 6 mg sodium

Rich Duck Stock

MAKES 6 CUPS

Of all the stocks we cover, this is the richest in flavor depth and can be used in many stews and casseroles, especially with poultry. It's a natural product of the two methods of cooking duck (see pp. 152–53).

INGREDIENTS

1 teaspoon	OLIVE OIL
2 cups	CHOPPED SWEET ONION
	DUCK NECK AND GIBLETS (if provided)
1	TRIMMED CARCASS (breast, legs removed)
8 cups	FILTERED WATER
2 teaspoons	SALT
1 Tablespoon	HERBS OF PROVENCE

BEFORE YOU COOK:

Heat medium saucepan. Chop the onion. Rinse the carcass and giblets well and then dry on paper towels.

COOKING METHOD

1. Pour oil into a heated saucepan. Add the onions and sauté till quite brown, stirring occasionally, 10 minutes.
2. Add giblets and carcass. Cover with water. Add salt and herbs.
3. Cover and bring to a boil. Reduce the heat to achieve an active simmer. Skim off surface foam occasionally. Cook one hour. Strain, remove surface fat, and cool in the refrigerator. See pages 152–54 for uses.

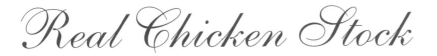
Real Chicken Stock
MAKES 2 1/2 CUPS

*One of the **real** reasons for buying a whole bird and roasting it is that you have more than one-third of its weight as bones to use for a delicious stock. With our **reduced** stock, we can upgrade many dishes, and it's virtually **free!***

INGREDIENTS

10–12 ounces	VEGETABLE TRIM (see p. 222)
1 pound	CHICKEN BONES
7 cups	WATER
1	BAY LEAF
2 teaspoons	HERBS OF PROVENCE (see p. 30, n. 8)
2 teaspoons	SALT

BEFORE YOU COOK:

Strip the chicken carcass of all usable meat, but leave all the fatty skin for the stock. Crush the carcass.

COOKING METHOD

1. Cover the crushed chicken and vegetable trim with 7 cups water. Add herbs and salt. Cover, bring to a boil, and reduce to a simmer with the lid on. Simmer 1 hour, skimming occasionally.
2. Strain off all solids and bring to a boil. Reduce by 50 percent to about 2 cups.
3. Skim off fat. Pour into an *old* ice cube tray and freeze.
4. When frozen, turn out cubes and store in a dated, freezer-quality zip-top bag in the freezer.

AT A GLANCE
(FOR SKILLED COOKS IN A HURRY)

Crush carcass. Add vegetable trim and cover with 7 cups water. Add herbs and salt. Boil, then simmer for 1 hour. Skim. Strain and reduce to 2 cups. Put in ice cube tray and freeze. Bag for future use.

Beef Stock

A great many fully prepared and/or "just add water" concentrates are available that provide a swift way to obtain "stock." All are better than tap water; some are very high in sodium. I prefer to adjust the seasoning of the entire dish, just before serving, so here is a method you can use on a quiet, cold winter's weekend. (Triple it—or more—and freeze for later on?)

INGREDIENTS

1 pound	BEEF BONES, fat trimmed off		1	BAY LEAF
1 teaspoon	NON-AROMATIC OLIVE OIL		1 teaspoon	DRIED THYME
1	ONION, coarsely chopped		6	BLACK PEPPERCORNS
½ cup	CELERY, coarsely chopped leaves and tops		2	WHOLE CLOVES
1 cup	CARROTS, coarsely chopped		8 cups	WATER

BEFORE YOU COOK!

Trim fat, chop onion, celery, and carrots, and measure the rest.

COOKING METHOD

1. Preheat the oven to 425°F. Place the beef bones in a roasting pan and cook until nicely browned, about 25 minutes. The browning produces a richer flavor and deeper color in the final stock.
2. Pour the oil into a large stock pot over medium heat. Add the onion, celery, and carrots and fry to release their volatile oils, about 5 minutes. Add the bones, bay leaf, thyme, pep-percorns, and cloves. Pour in the water, bring to a boil, reduce the heat, and simmer 4 to 8 hours, adding more water if necessary. Skim off any foam as it rises to the surface.
3. Pour through a fine strainer, discard the solids, and skim off all the fat. The stock can be frozen for up to 6 months.

NUTRITIONAL ANALYSIS

Per serving: 12 calories, 0 g carbohydrate, 0 g fat, 0 g saturated fat, 0% calories from saturated fat, 18 mg sodium, 0 g dietary fiber

AT A GLANCE
(FOR SKILLED COOKS IN A HURRY)

Preheat oven 425°F, roast to brown 25 minutes, sauté vegetables in oil 5 minutes. Add herbs, add water, boil, skim, reduce to simmer 4-8 hours. Strain, clear, freeze, or use.

Yogurt "Butter" Spread

We make this combination spread once a week. For several years we got used to the convenience of other low-fat spreads, but when we came back to our blend, it was such an improvement that we stayed with it. This is a spread only and can't be used for cooking.

INGREDIENTS

2 pound carton	PLAIN NONFAT YOGURT* (no starch or gelatin added)
1 pound carton	LOW-FAT VEGETABLE SPREAD** (no trans fats)

*Dannon does it well
**Such as "I Can't Believe It's Not Butter Light"

BEFORE YOU COOK:

Using a fine-mesh strainer or colander (see p. 38, n. 10). Line with paper towel and set over a bowl to catch 16 ounces (2 c.) of whey. Cover the sieve with a plate and refrigerate.

COOKING METHOD

1. Allow yogurt to drip for at least 12 hours (more won't harm it) in the refrigerator.
2. Discard the whey and mix the yogurt cheese with the low-fat vegetable spread until it turns an even pale color. Return it to the 2-pound container and store in the refrigerator (40°F).
3. Your spread will last 2 to 3 weeks.

NUTRITIONAL ANALYSIS

Per serving: 67 calories; 2 g protein; 2 g carbohydrates; 6 g fat; 1 g saturated fat; 113 mg sodium; 71 mg calcium; 0 mg iron; 101 RE Vitamin A; 1 mg Vitamin C; 0 mg Vitamin E; 0 g fiber

AT A GLANCE
(FOR SKILLED COOKS IN A HURRY)

Drain 2 pounds plain yogurt to get 1 pound (12 hrs. plus). Mix well with 1 pound low-fat vegetable spread. Use as needed.

Roasted Tomato Salsa

SERVES 4

I'm very grateful to the excellent "Rick Bayless's Mexican Kitchen" for this perfectly flavored tomato salsa. It's hot!

INGREDIENTS

1 pound	ITALIAN PLUM TOMATOES, such as Roma
2	FRESH JALAPEÑO PEPPERS
3 cloves	GARLIC, unpeeled
1/2 teaspoon	SALT
1/3 cup	SWEET ONION, finely chopped
1/2 cup	CILANTRO, loosely packed, chopped

COOKING METHOD

1. Preheat the broiler.
2. Line a shallow baking pan with aluminum foil and lay the whole tomatoes on it. Broil the tomatoes until their skins are blistered and blackened, about 6 minutes. Turn and blacken the other side. Cool and peel, reserving the juices.
3. Heat a heavy frying pan over medium heat. Lay the chiles and garlic in the dry pan and turn occasionally until soft, 5 to 10 minutes for the chiles and up to 15 minutes for the garlic. A quick pinch will tell you if they are ready. They should be softened and yield to slight pressure. Cool, peel the garlic, and remove the stem from the chiles.
4. Pulse the chiles, garlic, and salt in a blender or food processor. Add the tomatoes and their reserved juice and pulse a few times more, until coarsely chopped. Pour the mixture into a bowl, stir in the onion and cilantro, and set aside until ready to serve. This salsa will keep in the refrigerator for one or two days.

NUTRITIONAL ANALYSIS

Per serving: 42 calories; 1 g protein; 9 g carbohydrates; .5 g fat; 0 g saturated fat; 0% of calories from saturated fat; 157 mg sodium; 18 mg calcium; 1 mg iron; 129 RE Vitamin A; 26 mg Vitamin C; 1 mg Vitamin E; 2 g dietary fiber

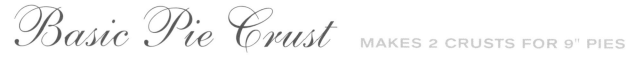

Basic Pie Crust

This pie crust is almost fool proof. It has a really good flavor, is crisp yet tender, and pairs beautifully with my crusted dishes.

INGREDIENTS

1 1/2 cups	CAKE FLOUR
1 teaspoon	SUGAR
1/8 teaspoon	SALT
2 Tablespoons	NONAROMATIC OLIVE OIL
1/4 cup	HARD MARGARINE OR BUTTER, frozen for 15 minutes
1 teaspoon	VINEGAR
4 Tablespoons	ICE WATER

METHOD OF ASSEMBLY

1. Combine the flour, sugar, and salt in a food processor. Pour in the oil, and pulse until mixed. Cut the margarine or butter into small pieces, and add to the flour mixture. Pulse 10 times or until the mixture is full of lumps the size of small peas.
2. Pour in the vinegar and ice water. Pulse 10 more times or until the dough begins to hold together. Gather into 2 equal balls, wrap separately, and refrigerate at least 30 minutes before rolling out.

Note: This dough can, of course, be made by hand. Combine the flour, sugar, and salt, and stir in the oil. Add the margarine, and mix with a pastry cutter or 2 knives until the size of small peas. Add the vinegar and ice water, and mix with a fork just until it starts to hold together. Gather into 2 balls, wrap, and refrigerate as above.

NUTRITIONAL ANALYSIS

Per serving: 78 calories, 5 g fat, 1 g saturated fat, 11% calories from saturated fat, 8 g carbohydrates, 0 g fiber, 52 mg. sodium

NIBBLES

Nibbles have now become a fixture in our new lifestyle for a lifetime. Once again please listen when I say "our choice for our lifestyle." Treena and I are now in our early seventies and have watched in fascination as our metabolism has gradually lessened. We have less need for the amount of food we once ate with gusto and burned off by leaping chairs (amongst other fringe lunatic pursuits!).

We now have more graceful adventures in movement and burn less. All this to say, we find that one hot, well-balanced, multiserving-of-vegetables-a-day meal is enough, and we prefer this at midday (if practical). When that happens we lighten-up for a supper with nibbles: an attractive plate of small-sized, flavor-filled "biteable" snacks that all contribute to our well-being without the empty-harm delivered by many "cultural snack foods."

Here are some examples from which you could select the ones that appeal to your taste. Make it up as an evening TV platter or as a side "dish" for scrabble or chess or simply as an exercise for a wandering hand during a page-turning novel by Ted Dekker.

- *Romaine lettuce* leaves lightly dressed in Treena's dressing (p. 84)
- *Cherry tomatoes* with a few small leaves of fresh basil
- *Watercress* (if available), also dressed as above
- *Low fat* (never nonfat) *cheese,* (Camembert or Monterey Jack, 8 oz. max)
- *Canadian bacon* (halved, 2 slices max)
- *Hard-boiled egg* (see p. 51), one only
- *Pear** (we like the brown BOSC), 1/2 each (cored and diced)
- *Apple** (we like Gala), 1/2 each (cored and diced)
- *Lean roasted meat* or poultry (we like lamb, 2 oz. max)
- *Raw vegetables:* snow peas, sugar snap peas, celery, green onion, radish, cucumber, carrot
- *Pickles,* olives, artichoke (pickled), beet root (watch the sodium)
- *Whole grain bread,* crackers, or crisp bread (usually not more than 1 slice)

We drink either water or a 3-4 oz. glass of Fre (see p. 32, n. 19). Sodas and soft drinks of all kinds—regardless of calories or sugars—no longer have a place in our lifestyle.

Now *please* imagine an attractive plate with a dozen or so "nibbles" of the ones *you* like. Wouldn't that be an interesting alternative to the cultural snacks that occupy our weight but seldom our *conscious* minds?

---

* We keep the use of fruit to a minimum because of Treena's diabetes. Berries are fine—blackberries and organic strawberries—but orange, pineapple, and dried fruits and grapes all tend to elevate her post prandial sugar (tested 2 hrs. after the first bite).

FRUIT ON FRUIT

You are now about to set sail on a sea of potential elegance. To my mind, palate, and experience, nothing beats the extraordinary delicacy of properly cooked, spiced, and partnered fruit.

For each of the twenty-seven different fruits, I've suggested the name of a good variety, when it's available on a national basis, and the season when it should be in ready supply. Also, I've included suggestions for cooking methods (which are more fully discussed at the end of the list) and the results of our experiments using Ariel de-alcoholized wines as a cooking medium. You may, of course, choose Ariel or wines with alcohol according to your personal preference. When alcohol is added to a dish, the number of calories will rise. The dessert with alcohol may not be suitable for, or enjoyed by, children, and the seasoning will need to be more robust in order to balance the alcohol "burn."

As of the date of publication, I need to explain that not all de-alcoholized wines are acceptable in these recipes because differ-ent production methods are used with vary-ing degrees of success. I use Ariel brand as my standard of quality.

I have also reviewed the world of spices and have suggested several that will react like nuclear fusion when *one plus one equals two point three.* The flavor combinations become more than the sum of the two ingre-dients and explode in your mouth! You will find sauce suggestions and will be able to select from your own basic recipes or mine, which follow.

Finally, I've listed companion fruits that you might like to present as a team. All in all, you have a *minimum* of five variations for each of the twenty-seven fruits, or at least 135 ideas!

However you choose to mix and match, you'll be reducing the health risks from the types of desserts that you literally have to die for! Here are the basic techniques to help you on your way. In every case the fruit des-serts can be served from pan to plate hot or allowed to cool and served chilled.

COOKING WITH FRUIT

FRUIT	VARIETY	JUN	JUL	AUG	SEP	OCT	NOV	DEC	JAN	FEB	MAR	APR	MAY	BRAISE	SAUTÉ	BAKE	ICE	SAUCE	POACH	LIQUID #1	LIQUID #2	SPICE #1	SPICE #2	COMPANION FRUITS	YOUR NOTES
APPLES - cooking	McIntosh	•	•	●	●	●	●	•	•	•	•	•	•	✓	✓	✓					Apple Juice	Cinnamon	Allspice	Cranberry, Rhubarb	
APRICOTS	Tilton	●	●	●	●										✓			✓	✓	White Zinfandel		Cardamom	Cloves	Papaya, Pineapple	
ASIAN PEARS (Nashi)	20th Century			●	●	●	●												✓	White Wine		Allspice	Cinnamon	Banana, Mango	
BANANAS	Cavendish	●	●	●	●	●	●	●	●	●	●	●	●		✓					White Zinfandel		Allspice	Cardamom	Raspberry, Pineapple	
BLACKBERRIES	Ollalie	●	●	●	●												✓	✓		White Wine		Cinnamon	Ginger	Other berries, Cranberry	
BLUEBERRIES	Bluecrop	●	●	●														✓		White Wine		Cinnamon	Ginger	Other berries, Cranberry	
CHERRIES	Rainer	●	●											✓				✓	✓	Champagne	White Wine	Cardamom	Ginger	Orange, Banana	
CRANBERRIES	McFarlin					●	●	●						✓			✓			White Zinfandel	Apple Juice	Cinnamon	Ginger	Oranges, Green Grapes	
DATES	Deglet Noor			●	●	●	●	●	●	●									✓	White Zinfandel		Ginger	Allspice	Mango, Orange	
FIGS	White Kadota			●	●	●											✓			White Wine		Allspice	Cinnamon	Apricot, Mango	
GRAPEFRUIT	Texas Pink							●	●	●	●	●								White Wine	Champagne	Mint		Strawberries, Grapes	
GRAPES	Thompson seedless		●	●	•	•	•	•	•	•	•								✓	White Wine	Champagne	Cinnamon	Ginger	Kiwi, Mango	
KIWIFRUIT	Hayward	●	●			●	●	●	●	●	●	●	●							Blanc	Champagne	Allspice	Cardamom	Mango, Banana	
LYCHEES	Brewster	●	●																✓	White Wine	Champagne	Ginger	Cardamom	Asian pear, Papaya	

Dots indicate availability but not in prime season (and sometimes transported long distances)

COOKING WITH FRUIT

FRUIT	VARIETY	JUN	JUL	AUG	SEP	OCT	NOV	DEC	JAN	FEB	MAR	APR	MAY	BRAISE	SAUTE'	BAKE	ICE	SAUCE	POACH	LIQUID #1	LIQUID #2	SPICE #1	SPICE #2	COMPANION FRUITS	YOUR NOTES
MANGOES	Tommy Atkins	■	■									■	■	✓				✓		White Wine	Champagne	Cardamom	Nutmeg	Papaya, Pineapple	
MELONS	Cantaloupe			■	■	■													✓	White Wine	Champagne	Cardamom	Nutmeg	Kiwi, Grapes	
NECTARINES	Summer Grand					■						■	■					✓		White Wine		Nutmeg	Allspice	Banana, Raspberry	
ORANGES	Navel						■	■	■	■	■						✓			White Zinfandel		Mint		Grapes, Nectarines	
PAPAYAS	Solo	•	•	•	•	•	•	•	•	•	•	•						✓	✓	White Wine	Champagne	Cinnamon	Cardamom	Banana, Strawberry	
PEACHES	Redhaven	•		■	•								•			✓	✓			White Wine	Champagne	Allspice	Cinnamon	Apricots, Raspberries	
PEARS	Bosc					■	■	■	■	■	■			✓		✓	✓		✓	White Wine	Champagne	Ginger	Cinnamon	Cranberry, Apricot	
PINEAPPLES	Sugar Loaf	•	•	•	•	•	•	•	•	•	•			✓			✓	✓		White Wine	White Zinfandel	Cardamom	Ginger	Grapes, Blueberries, Apricots	
PLUMS	Santa Rosa	■	■	■	■							■	■					✓		White Wine		Cardamom	Cinnamon	Blackberries, Pears	
PRUNES	d'Agen Prune		■	■	■	■	■	■	■	■	■						✓	✓	✓	White Wine		Cinnamon	Ginger	Apple, Asian Pear	
RASPBERRIES	Meeker																✓	✓		White Wine		Cardamom	Cinnamon	Other berries, Mango	
RHUBARB	Crimson Rhubarb											■	■	✓			✓	✓		White Zinfandel	Champagne	Cinnamon	Mint	Blueberry, Orange	
STRAWBERRIES	Selva	■	■														✓	✓		White Wine		Cinnamon		Rhubarb, Dates, Other berries	

Dots indicate availability but not in prime season (and sometimes transported long distances)

BASIC FRUIT PREPARATION METHODS

SAUTE The oil should be neutral in flavor, such as the extra light (refers to flavor) flavorless olive oil. Then you can add a few drops of toasted sesame seed oil for a nutty flavor. I use very little—one teaspoonful of oil for a four-portion dessert.

Heat the oil in a skillet and add fruit that has been cut into 1-inch-thick slices or wedges. Sprinkle with a little ground spice, using no more than 1/16 teaspoon per panful of fruit and 1 tablespoon of sugar (depending on the fruit to be served, of course).

Set on a moderate heat to steam through and let the sweet juices mingle and caramelize when sufficiently concentrated. Serve these simple sautés with frozen low-fat yogurt spooned over a slice of angel food cake, or wrapped in a thin pancake or crêpe.

POACH When poaching, you must rely upon a beautifully seasoned pool of cooking liquid being brought up to the boil while never being allowed to actually bubble. In this hot bath, the fruit will gently relax as the internal temperatures rise and force the natural juices out to mingle with the hot liquid. When the heat is turned down, the juices return to the fruit and the miracle of multiplied flavors begins.

The poaching liquid can be totally or partly created from wine or clear fruit juices, or a blend. My personal preference is to use de-alcoholized wines, and I recommend Ariel brands. Finely grated citrus zests (orange, grapefruit, lime, tangerine) can be added to the liquid but, for my taste, must be removed before serving.

When the peeled and sliced fruit is perfectly cooked, lift it from the liquid and keep it warm. Strain the liquid and return it to a saucepan to be thickened with a little cornstarch or arrowroot (1 Tbsp. to each 1 c. of liquid) mixed first into a slurry with cold juices. Bring the sauce to a boil for 30 seconds to clear the starchy taste of the cornstarch (this is unnecessary when using arrowroot).

Please try it then, and add a little sugar or freshly squeezed lemon juice according to taste, and *maybe* a touch more of a warm, aromatic spice such as cloves, cinnamon, nutmeg, allspice, or cardamom. Coat the fruit with the sauce and serve it hot over cold rice pudding or just as it is.

BROIL (radiant overhead heat) Peel and core or pit the fruit and brush lightly with melted brown sugar, seasoned to your liking with warming spices. Place on a nonstick baking pan so that the tops of the fruit are about 4 inches from the heat source. Cook until just lightly browned.

I like to serve broiled fruit with a sprig of cool, fresh green mint and wedges of orange or lemon on the side, with perhaps a couple of gingersnap cookies.

BAKE This method produces much the same result as broiling, but obviously takes a little longer and permits larger pieces to be more evenly cooked. It has the added benefit of not having to be watched all the time.

Oven temperatures should be 350°F for juicy fruit and 425°F for apricots, pears, and peaches. Baking times run from 30 minutes down to 20 minutes for fruit with a higher sugar content.

A baste can be made with reduced de-alcoholized wine, brown sugar, and one of the warming spices. As always, please be restrained with the amount of spice added.

BRAISE This is a poaching process that takes place in the oven. The fruit is almost covered with the poaching liquid and baked at 350°F for 30 minutes or until tender. As with poaching, the juices can be thickened and warmly seasoned to taste.

SMOOTH SAUCES All fruit can be made into smooth sauces. Some need an extra sieving to eliminate seeds or fiber, but otherwise all can be poached until very tender and then puréed (whizzed) in a blender along with a small amount of the cooking liquid.

A simple fine mesh and a wooden spoon will help to swiftly strain seeds and fiber.

In some cases you may need to add a little arrowroot slurry, one tablespoon for each one cup of liquid. Arrowroot brings a brilliantly clear gloss to the sauce and seems to brighten the color without obscuring the taste.

Please buy arrowroot by the one-pound packet in a health food store or food cooperative and not in small, expensive glass jars.

For custard-style sauces that are low in fat and calories, all you need to do is gently stir in low-fat vanilla yogurt. You can also blend dense poached fruit such as pears, bananas, apples, apricots, or peaches with unsweetened evaporated skim milk in the ratio of 8 fluid ounces (1 c.) for each 1 pound of fruit and sweeten to taste.

MACERATE This is an almost out-of-date term that needs to be revived. It comes from the French *maceérer,* to place fruit in a liquid to absorb or give off flavor. I macerate fruit in de-alcoholized wines that I have reduced by half in order to concentrate their flavor. After the fruit has soaked overnight, I take a third of the volume and sieve it to produce a purée. I use this as a sauce for the remaining macerated fruit.

FRUIT ICES Many of the fruits mentioned can be made into a frozen dessert. You can make a triple batch when poaching, baking, braising, or shallow frying and let the fruit cool in its extra cooking juices. Whiz it in a blender until smooth, pour into a tray, and partially freeze. Then whip the slush to beat air into it and return to the freezer.

You can use this same fruit purée in an ice cream machine with really excellent results.

EXAMPLE:

FOOD, ETC.	SIZE	CALS	FAT	CARBS	ESTIMATED DAILY/WEEKLY CONSUMED	DECISION R/M	UNIT SAVINGS	WKLY CALS	WKLY FAT	WKLY CARBS	COST SAVINGS DAILY/WEEKLY: ANNUAL
COOKIES											
Chocolate chip	1 oz.	110	6	15							
Biscotti	1 oz.	130	5	20							
Low fat Oatmeal	1 oz.	90	0	20	1 2 3 4 5 (6)	4	2	180	0	40	20¢ x 2 = 40¢: $146 per year
COLA											
	8 oz.	100	0	25							
	12 oz.	150	0	37	1 2 3 (4) 5	2 x 12 oz.	2 x 12 oz.	300	0	74	2 x 12 oz = $2: $255 per year
	16 oz.	250	0	63							
	Diet	0	0	0							
POTATO CHIPS											
	1 oz.	150	10	15							
	4 oz.	600	40	60	(1) 2 3	1 x lowfat	(diff)	40	8.5	<8>	Nil
Lowfat baked	1 oz.	110	1.5	23							
STEAK											
	3 oz.	195	10	0	3 oz. 5 oz. (8 oz.) (x per week = 3)	3 x 5 oz.	9 oz.	540	30	0	$.5 - $240 per year
	5 oz.	400	20	0							
	8 oz.	520	26	0							

These four examples show how we did our assessments.

Cookies: We buy lowfat oatmeal (1 oz.) and used to eat 6 per day. (We put parenthesis around 6). Under R/M (reasonable moderate) we cut back to 2 each = 4. We then had a savings of 2. We multiplied the weekly nutrition values x 2 = 180 / 0 / 40 and put in our cost savings 20¢ each = 40¢ per day x 365 = $146 a year!

Colas: We used to buy 4 colas a day (12 oz.). We decided on one each. (We saved 2 x 12 oz.) – our weekly nutrition savings were 300 / 0 / 74, and cost savings of 2 x 80¢ = $1.60 x 365 = $255 a year.

Potato Chips: We used to have a 1 oz. packet each once or twice a week. We now buy lowfat baked, say 2 per week, at the same price. Therefore it's only a nutrition difference between regular and lowfat baked, or (80 / 17 / <16>). *NOTE:* the carbs go up, so we put them within arrows.

Steak: We used to have an 8 oz. steak (chop) etc., 3 times a week. We decided our R/M would be 3 oz. (cooked weight) and so we saved 3 x 5 oz. – 15 oz. a week – 780 oz. per year (48 lbs. @ $5 per lb. = $240). The weekly nutrition "savings" (540/30/0) is about 8 lbs. of body fat weight loss per year and reduced risk from saturated fat.

FAVORITE FOODS

	FOOD, ETC.	SIZE	CALS	FAT	CARBS	ESTIMATED DAILY/WEEKLY CONSUMED	DECISION R/M	UNIT SAVINGS	WKLY CALS	WKLY FAT	WKLY CARBS	COST SAVINGS DAILY/WEEKLY: ANNUAL
1.	**Whole milk**	1 cup	150	8	12							
	2%		130	5	13							
	Skim		90	5	13							
2.	**Silk (Soy) Vanilla**		100	3.5	10							
3.	**Plain yogurt**	1 cup	180	7	11							
	Lowfat		140	4	16							
	Non-fat		110	0	18							
	+Fruit (whole)		250	6	38							
	+Fruit (lowfat)		230	3	32							
	+Fruit (nonfat)		150	0	32							
	(no sugar added)		120	0	32							
4.	**Ice Cream**	½ cup										
	Reg 10%		130	7	16							
	16%		170	10	17							
	20%		270	18	21							
	6%		140	4	18							
	<4%		120	2.5	22							
	Fat Free		100	0	22							
	Soft serve nonfat		90	0	23							
	Frozen yogurt nonfat		110	0	29							
	Waffle cones		60	100	22							
	Waffle cones		20	40								

FAVORITE FOODS

FOOD, ETC.	SIZE	CALS	FAT	CARBS	ESTIMATED DAILY/WEEKLY CONSUMED	DECISION R/M	UNIT SAVINGS	WKLY CALS	WKLY FAT	WKLY CARBS	COST SAVINGS DAILY/WEEKLY: ANNUAL
5. Creams	1 Tbsp.										
Half and half		20	2	.5							
Light (20%)		30	3	.5							
Med (25%)		20	2	.5							
Sour		30	3	.5							
Whipping cream (37%)	2 Tbsp. whipped	50	5	1							
Lite (30%)		45	4.5	.5							
Coconut cream	¼ cup	90	9	1							
Premium		125	12	3							
Cool Whip Free	2 Tbsp.	15	0	3							
Lite		20	1	2							
Coffee creamer flavored & fat free	1 1/3 Tbsp.	50	0	11							
6. Butter (reg.)	1 Tbsp.	100	11	0							
Whipped (reg.)	1 tsp.	70	7.5	0							
Whipped (light 40%)		35	3.5	0							
C.B.I.B. (reg.)	1 Tbsp.	90	10	0							
C.B.I.B. (lite)		50	6	0							
Land O' Lakes (lite whipped)		35	3.5	0							
Brummel Brown		45	5	0							
7. Mayonnaise (reg.)	1 Tbsp.	100	11	.5							
(lite)		50	5	1							
8. Vegetable oil	1 Tbsp.	120	14	0							
Vegetable shortening		113	13	0							

FAVORITE FOODS

FOOD, ETC.	SIZE	CALS	FAT	CARBS	ESTIMATED DAILY/WEEKLY CONSUMED	DECISION R/M	UNIT SAVINGS	WKLY CALS	WKLY FAT	WKLY CARBS	COST SAVINGS DAILY/WEEKLY: ANNUAL
9. Lard, etc.		115	13	0							
Chee		110	13	0							
10. Cheese (hard)	1 oz. piece	110	9	.5							
Grated	1 Tbsp.	27	2	0							
Grated	¼ cup	110	9	.5							
Light	1 oz.	80	5	.5							
Fat free	1 oz.	50	0	2							
11. Eggs (whole)	50 g.	75	4.5	0							
Egg Beaters	¼ cup	30	0	0							
12. Steak (w/fat)	3 oz. (4.5 oz.)	230	14	0							
Lean & marbling		195	10	0							
Lean (5 oz.)		400	20	0							
Lean (8 oz.)		520	26	0							
Lean (12 oz.)		780	39	0							
Lamb chop	2 ¼-4 ¼	200	15	0							
Pork chop	3 oz.	200	11	0							
13. Bacon (raw) med. slice	¾	125	13	0							
Cooked, 1 slice	6 g.	36	3	0							
Cooked, thick	12 g.	70	6	0							
Canadian bacon	1 oz.	45	4	1							
Ham (reg.) 11% fat	1 oz.	52	3	0							
5% fat		37	2	0							

FAVORITE FOODS

	FOOD, ETC.	SIZE	CALS	FAT	CARBS	ESTIMATED DAILY/WEEKLY CONSUMED	DECISION R/M	UNIT SAVINGS	WKLY CALS	WKLY FAT	WKLY CARBS	COST SAVINGS DAILY/WEEKLY: ANNUAL
14.	**Game** Buffalo	4 oz.	70	3	0							
	Venison	3 oz.	135	3	0							
	Ostrich	4 oz.	130	2.5	0							
	Rabbit	3 oz.	130	14	0							
	Liver	3 oz.	200	9	0							
15.	**Sausage** (cooked) med.	2 oz.	100	8	2.5							
	Large	3 oz.	150	12	3.5							
	Italian (cooked)	2-4	215	17	1.5							
	Chorza, raw	2.5	320	31	3							
16.	**Chicken Roast** w/o skin	4 oz.	215	8	0							
	plus skin & fat	4 oz.	270	15								
	Batter fried		330	20	11							
	Drumstick (w/o skin)	1 ½ oz.	125 (75)	6 (2)	0							
17.	**Pizza 12" reg.**	¼	350	14	36							
	+ cheese		380	16	40							
	Celebrity styled		410	20	60							
18.	**Salad dressings**	2 Tbsp.										
	Blue Cheese		150	16	2							
	Lite		80	8	1							
	Caesar		140	14	2							
	Lite		50	5	.5							
	Italian		130	11	3							
	Lite		70	7	2							
	Ranch		160	18	3							
	Lite		90	8	3							
	1000 Island		130	12	5							
	Lite		50	4	3							

FAVORITE FOODS

	FOOD, ETC.	SIZE	CALS	FAT	CARBS	ESTIMATED DAILY/WEEKLY CONSUMED	DECISION R/M	UNIT SAVINGS	WKLY CALS	WKLY FAT	WKLY CARBS	COST SAVINGS DAILY/WEEKLY: ANNUAL
19.	**Cereals**											
	Oatmeal (cooked)	1 cup	145	3	25							
		6 oz.	110	2	19							
	Raisin Bran Crunch (2 oz.)	1 cup	190	1	44							
20.	**Breads**											
	Toast, slice	1.2 oz.	85	1	16							
	Thick	1.5 oz.	105	1.5	20							
	Bagels	2 oz.	160	1.5	30							
		4 oz.	320	3	60							
	Cream cheese	1 oz.	80	8	2							
	Reduced fat		60	5	2							
21.	**Cookies**											
	Biscotti	1 oz.	130	5	20							
	Chocolate chip	1 oz.	110	6	15							
	Oatmeal	1 oz.	95	3.5	15							
	Peanut butter	1 oz.	125	6.5	14							
	Lowfat choc. chip	1 oz.	100	1	21							
	Oatmeal low fat	1 oz.	90	0	20							
	Peanut butter	1 oz.	105	2	14							
22.	**Muffins** small	1 oz.	80	3	12							
		2 oz.	160	6	24							
		3 oz.	240	9	36							
		4 oz.	320	12	48							
		6 oz.	480	18	60							
		8 oz.	640	24	96							
	English muffins	2 oz.	150	2	29							
23.	**Donuts**	1 ¾ oz.	210	12	25							
	Glazed	2 oz.	250	12	34							

FAVORITE FOODS

	FOOD, ETC.	SIZE	CALS	FAT	CARBS	ESTIMATED DAILY/WEEKLY CONSUMED	DECISION R/M	UNIT SAVINGS	WKLY CALS	WKLY FAT	WKLY CARBS	COST SAVINGS DAILY/WEEKLY: ANNUAL
24.	**Pies** 1/8 of a 9-inch pie											
	Apple	4 oz.	290	13	46							
	Pecan	4 oz.	470	24	52							
	Pumpkin	4 oz.	240	13	28							
25.	**Pancakes**	3 inch	50	2.5	6							
		4 inch	80	3	11							
		5 inch	160	6	21							
	Syrup	1 Tbsp.	50	0	13							
	Butter	1 Tbsp.	70	7.5	0							
	1 x 5 inch + syrup/butter		280	13.5	34							
26.	**Waffles**	7 inch	245	15	26							
27.	**Sugars**	1 tsp.. (4 g.)	15	0	4							
	1 heaping teaspoon	6 g.	25	0	6.5							
	1 packet		25	0	6.5							
	Honey	1 tsp.	22	0	5.5							
	Jams	1 tsp.	18	0	5							
28.	**Chocolate** average	1 oz.	150	10	13							
		2 oz.	300	20	30							
		4 oz.	600	40	60							
29.	**Potato Chips**	1 chip	9	1	1							
	1 oz. pkg	17 chips	150	10	15							
	4 oz. pkg		600	40	60							
	Lowfat baked	1 oz.	110	1.5	23							
	Corn chips	1 oz.	160	10	15							
	Tortilla chips	15 chips	150	8	22							

FAVORITE FOODS

	FOOD, ETC.	SIZE	CALS	FAT	CARBS	ESTIMATED DAILY/WEEKLY CONSUMED	DECISION R/M	UNIT SAVINGS	WKLY CALS	WKLY FAT	WKLY CARBS	COST SAVINGS DAILY/WEEKLY: ANNUAL
30.	**Nuts** (*nuts per 1 oz.) Walnuts (18)	1 oz.	175	16	3.5							
	Pecans (20)	1 oz.	190	19	5							
	Macadamia (10)	1 oz.	200	21	4							
	Hazelnut (18-20)	1 oz.	180	18	4.5							
	Cashews (18)	1 oz.	165	14	10							
	Brazil (8)	1 oz.	185	19	3.5							
	Almonds (24-28)	1 oz.	170	15	7							
	Pumpkin seeds	1 oz.	155	13	5							
	Peanut butter spread	1 tsp.	35	3	1.5							
31.	**Potatoes**	2 oz.	45	0	11							
		3 oz.	65	0	15							
		5 oz.	110	0	26							
	Baked + skins	7 oz.	220	0	51							
	Mashed + milk	½ cup	110	4	14							
	Hash browns	½ cup	165	10	10							
	French fries	2.5 oz.	220	12	14							
	French fries	4 oz.	350	20	22							
	McDonald's (supersize)	7 oz.	610	29	77							
	Potato salad, ½ cup	4 ¼ oz.	180	10	14							
32.	**Rice** (1/2 cup)	3 ¼ oz.										
	Short Grain, boiled		120	0	27							
	Long Grain, boiled		100	0	22							
	Brown, boiled		110	.05	23							
33.	**Pasta**											
	(1 oz. dry= 2.5-3 oz. cooked)	2 oz. dry	210	1	42							
34.	**Bread rolls**											
	med. 3 inch diameter	1 ½ oz.	130	3	23							

FAVORITE FOODS

FOOD, ETC.	SIZE	CALS	FAT	CARBS	ESTIMATED DAILY/WEEKLY CONSUMED	DECISION R/M	UNIT SAVINGS	WKLY CALS	WKLY FAT	WKLY CARBS	COST SAVINGS DAILY/WEEKLY: ANNUAL
35.											
Beverages											
Orange juice ½ cup	4 oz.	55	0	13							
	6 oz.	82	0	20							
	8 oz.	110	0	26							
Cola	8 oz.	100	0	25							
	12 oz.	150	0	37							
	16 oz.	200	0	50							
	20 oz.	250	0	63							
Iced tea (sweet)	8 oz.	100	0	25							
	12 oz.	150	0	38							
(unsweetened)	8 oz.	2	0	0							
Beer (5%)	7 oz.	80	8.5	4							
	12 oz.	140	14	10							
Beer (4.2%)	7 oz.	65	7	4							
	12 oz.	110	12	7							
Beer (DA)*	12 oz.	70	1	16							
Wine (11.5%)	4 oz.	85	11	2							
	6 oz.	125	16	3							
(dry)	4 oz.	50	0	12							
Spirits 40% 80 proof	1 oz.	65	9.5	0							
Spirits 43% 86 proof	1 oz.	70	10	0							
Spirits 50% 100 proof	1 oz.	82	12	0							

*without alcohol

Body Mass Index Table

	Normal						Overweight					Obese										Extreme Obesity														
BMI	19	20	21	22	23	24	25	26	27	28	29	30	31	32	33	34	35	36	37	38	39	40	41	42	43	44	45	46	47	48	49	50	51	52	53	54
Height (inches)												Body Weight (pounds)																								
58	91	96	100	105	110	115	119	124	129	134	138	143	148	153	158	162	167	172	177	181	186	191	196	201	205	210	215	220	224	229	234	239	244	248	253	258
59	94	99	104	109	114	119	124	128	133	138	143	148	153	158	163	168	173	178	183	188	193	198	203	208	212	217	222	227	232	237	242	247	252	257	262	267
60	97	102	107	112	118	123	128	133	138	143	148	153	158	163	168	174	179	184	189	194	199	204	209	215	220	225	230	235	240	245	250	255	261	266	271	276
61	100	106	111	116	122	127	132	137	143	148	153	158	164	169	174	180	185	190	195	201	206	211	217	222	227	232	238	243	248	254	259	264	269	275	280	285
62	104	109	115	120	126	131	136	142	147	153	158	164	169	175	180	186	191	196	202	207	213	218	224	229	235	240	246	251	256	262	267	273	278	284	289	295
63	107	113	118	124	130	135	141	146	152	158	163	169	175	180	186	191	197	203	208	214	220	225	231	237	242	248	254	259	265	270	278	282	287	293	299	304
64	110	116	122	128	134	140	145	151	157	163	169	174	180	186	192	197	204	209	215	221	227	232	238	244	250	256	262	267	273	279	285	291	296	302	308	314
65	114	120	126	132	138	144	150	156	162	168	174	180	186	192	198	204	210	216	222	228	234	240	246	252	258	264	270	276	282	288	294	300	306	312	318	324
66	118	124	130	136	142	148	155	161	167	173	179	186	192	198	204	210	216	223	229	235	241	247	253	260	266	272	278	284	291	297	303	309	315	322	328	334
67	121	127	134	140	146	153	159	166	172	178	185	191	198	204	211	217	223	230	236	242	249	255	261	268	274	280	287	293	299	306	312	319	325	331	338	344
68	125	131	138	144	151	158	164	171	177	184	190	197	203	210	216	223	230	236	243	249	256	262	269	276	282	289	295	302	308	315	322	328	335	341	348	354
69	128	135	142	149	155	162	169	176	182	189	196	203	209	216	223	230	236	243	250	257	263	270	277	284	291	297	304	311	318	324	331	338	345	351	358	365
70	132	139	146	153	160	167	174	181	188	195	202	209	216	222	229	236	243	250	257	264	271	278	285	292	299	306	313	320	327	334	341	348	355	362	369	376
71	136	143	150	157	165	172	179	186	193	200	208	215	222	229	236	243	250	257	265	272	279	286	293	301	308	315	322	329	338	343	351	358	365	372	379	386
72	140	147	154	162	169	177	184	191	199	206	213	221	228	235	242	250	258	265	272	279	287	294	302	309	316	324	331	338	346	353	361	368	375	383	390	397
73	144	151	159	166	174	182	189	197	204	212	219	227	235	242	250	257	265	272	280	288	295	302	310	318	325	333	340	348	355	363	371	378	386	393	401	408
74	148	155	163	171	179	186	194	202	210	218	225	233	241	249	256	264	272	280	287	295	303	311	319	326	334	342	350	358	365	373	381	389	396	404	412	420
75	152	160	168	176	184	192	200	208	216	224	232	240	248	256	264	272	279	287	295	303	311	319	327	335	343	351	359	367	375	383	391	399	407	415	423	431
76	156	164	172	180	189	197	205	213	221	230	238	246	254	263	271	279	287	295	304	312	320	328	336	344	353	361	369	377	385	394	402	410	418	426	435	443

Source: Adapted from *Clinical Guidelines on the Identification, Evaluation, and Treatment of Overweight and Obesity in Adults: The Evidence Report.*

REMARKS

Author's Notes

(A) Insert present average weight. Take each a.m. before eating. Average is your dotted line. Go up in 1 lb. and down in 1 lb. levels. Insert these numbers.

(B) If you are diabetic, use dotted line as your fasting upper level goal (i.e., 120 or 130). Go up-and-down in 10s. Insert these numbers.

(C) If you are hypertensive (or watching stress levels), use a "cuff" gauge like the Omron and record same time each day to spot trends.

(D) Steps: If you are counting steps, insert here your total from pedometer— you might have friendly competition with spouse or loved one/friend.

Fruits and Vegetables: Goal–5 to 9 servings a day. Insert your consumption.

Temperature: Not really necessary (I keep it to see how seasons affect our choices.).

	1	2	3	4	5	6	7	8	9	10	11	12	13	14	15	16	17	18	19	20	21	22	23	24	25	26	27	28	29	30	31	#
MORNING WEIGHT																																
(A) +																																
FASTING GLUCOSE (●) POST PRANDIAL ($\overline{\wedge}\ \underline{\vee}$)																																
(B)																																
SYSTOLIC BP (GOAL LESS THAN 130)																																
(C)																																
DIASTOLIC BP (GOAL LESS THAN 80)																																
(C)																																
RANDOM FACTORS																																
(D) Steps																																
Steps																																
Fruit/Veg																																
Temp.																																

	1	2	3	4	5	6	7	8	9	10	11	12	13	14	15	16	17	18	19	20	21	22	23	24	25	26	27	28	29	30	31	#

MORNING WEIGHT

(A)

FASTING GLUCOSE (•) POST PRANDIAL ($\overline{\wedge}^{\vee}$)

(B)

SYSTOLIC BP (GOAL LESS THAN 130)

(C)

DIASTOLIC BP (GOAL LESS THAN 80)

(C)

RANDOM FACTORS

(D)

Steps
Steps
Fruit/Veg
Temp.

FRUIT OF THE SPIRIT CHECKLIST

Here is the little list of qualities . . . really our general feelings about our life and how we are living it in our heads and hearts. You can complete it in now and then check it later in the year. It's such fun to see progress! Simply check the number after the feelings that best describe how you feel *TODAY*.

I'M GRATEFUL FOR THESE									
Love	1	2	3	4	5	6	7	8	9	10
Joy	1	2	3	4	5	6	7	8	9	10
Peace	1	2	3	4	5	6	7	8	9	10
Patience	1	2	3	4	5	6	7	8	9	10
Goodness	1	2	3	4	5	6	7	8	9	10
Kindness	1	2	3	4	5	6	7	8	9	10
Faithfulness	1	2	3	4	5	6	7	8	9	10
Gentleness	1	2	3	4	5	6	7	8	9	10
Self-control	1	2	3	4	5	6	7	8	9	10

I'M WORKING ON THESE									
Resentment	1	2	3	4	5	6	7	8	9	10
Despondent	1	2	3	4	5	6	7	8	9	10
Argumentative	1	2	3	4	5	6	7	8	9	10
Impatient	1	2	3	4	5	6	7	8	9	10
Impetuous	1	2	3	4	5	6	7	8	9	10
Abusive (Hurtful)	1	2	3	4	5	6	7	8	9	10
Unreliable	1	2	3	4	5	6	7	8	9	10
Conceited (Vain)	1	2	3	4	5	6	7	8	9	10
Dissatisfied	1	2	3	4	5	6	7	8	9	10

THE FOOD PREFERENCE SHEETS (FPS)

What you now have in your hands is the opportunity of a lifetime, and it really is your *lifetime* (and those you love)!

The FPS lists have morphed their way from November 1985 until today and will doubtless continue to be refined by practical experience . . . including yours perhaps?

You will need about one hour to complete the list in order to get it *right,* and if you spend that hour, it will provide you with a magnificent return. You will have a kind of MRI of your food memory. It will remind you about what you like, what you can accept, what you don't like, and what you haven't yet eaten.

From this list you will see *at a glance* all the foods you like and can accept—that's your preference; it's what you can eat often and enjoy.

Almost all of us enjoy certain foods as a treat, and that's part of the good life. Our problem lies when we increase the volume (amount) of the treat, and it becomes (by its very size) a threat. Most of us really do know where our weakness for large treats lies: the doughnut, the large latte, the double-scoop ice cream, that "splendid cheese," the chocolate cake (and the second slice), a heaping of smothered pasta with a cheese sauce. O my, but the list can be long. *I know;* we've been there!

So how to use the FPS to return to a treat . . .

1. When you've finished the list (you can make copies for your family to complete or they could do it free on www.graham kerr.com), go through it marking clearly your possible threats and putting in the amount you usually consume, i.e. double-scoop ice cream, large french fries, 16-ounce cola, 2-ounce cheese, 4-ounce chocolate, and so forth.

2. Now consider reducing your threats to treat size—i.e. single scoop, small fries, 8-ounce cola, 1-ounce cheese, 2-ounce chocolate—and insert that amount alongside your present consumption.

3. To fill the space left by the smaller amount, consider what could take its place (if needed). Go down your LIKE list and I *know* you'll find something that you will enjoy and that will also enhance your health (and also the wellness of those you love).

And now . . . how can the FPS help to change a recipe?

You may remember me in my earlier days as the Galloping Gourmet. My primary concern was from the neck up. In other words a recipe had to deliver a knock out blow to the senses. If the sensuality caused a threat to the rest of the body, well . . . that was some-one else's problem, not mine.

As a result the butter fat content (clari-fied butter) was usually 1/4 cup (2 oz.) for 4 people. Meat was averaged at 8 ounces a head. Salt was as much as it took (who mea-sures?!). My desserts overflowed with sugars and cream, and seldom was a vegetable more than a garnish!

For an occasional gourmet, I suppose it might work out, but for a day-to-day gourmet it would be off the charts!

So when one reduces meat, fat, sugar, and refined carbohydrates, there must be a replacement that delivers an enjoyable level of taste, aroma, color, and texture. This is why the FPS is split up into these four main sensory elements.

When you've identified a need to lessen an ingredient, please go over your FPS lists and find a replacement that appeals to your (or your loved ones') preferences.

It really will be according to *your* prefer-ences (not mine), and who knows . . . you may take out a favorite of mine and insert one of yours and all of a sudden you've cre-ated something new. It's fun, it's creative, it's individual, it's a healthy change . . . and it's *all* yours.

FOOD PREFERENCE SHEET

#1 SALT	LIKE IT	ACCEPTABLE	DON'T LIKE	DON'T KNOW
Anchovies				
Vegemite/Marmite				
Potato chips				
Tortilla chips				
Nuts				
Bacon				
Soy sauce (low sodium)				
Fish sauce (Asian)				
Capers				
Pickles				
Worcestershire sauce				
French fries				
Parmesan cheese				
Canadian bacon				
Ham hocks				
Prosciutto				
Smoked salmon				
Salami				
Chutneys				
Ham				
Lox				
Cheeses				
Pretzels				
Corned beef				
Rotisserie chicken				
Canned soups				
Canned sauces				
Packaged soups				
Packaged sauces				
Olives				
Smoked turkey				

#1 SALT CONTINUED	LIKE IT	ACCEPTABLE	DON'T LIKE IT	DON'T KNOW
Celery				
#2 SOUR	**LIKE IT**	**ACCEPTABLE**	**DON'T LIKE IT**	**DON'T KNOW**
Lemon				
Vinegar, malt				
Vinegar, white wine/cider				
Vinegar, red wine				
Pickles				
Capers				
Vinegar, balsamic				
Lime				
Vinegar, Rice				
Quince				
Beets, pickled				
Dijon mustard, etc.				
Ketchup				
Rhubarb				
Raspberries				
Strawberries				
Pineapple				
Kiwi Fruit				
Apples				
Cherries				
Tangerines				
Oranges				
Nectarines				
Peaches				
Apricots				
Blackberries				
Blueberries				
Seville marmalade				
Mayonnaise				

FOOD PREFERENCE SHEET

#2 SOUR CONTINUED	LIKE IT	ACCEPTABLE	DON'T LIKE IT	DON'T KNOW
Cranberries (unsweetened)				
Tomatillos				
#3 SWEET	**LIKE IT**	**ACCEPTABLE**	**DON'T LIKE IT**	**DON'T KNOW**
Honey				
White sugar				
Hard candy				
Candy bars				
Brown sugar				
Maple syrup				
Corn syrup				
Coffee flavored syrups				
Chocolate syrup				
Chocolate				
Molasses				
Glazed ginger				
Cookies				
Glazed doughnuts				
Frosted cake				
Sweetened condensed milk				
Jams				
Jellies				
Coconut (sweetened)				
Colas				
Doughnuts				
Cake				
Cold cereal				
Raisins				
Dates				
Cranberries (sweetened)				
Dried fruit				
Preserves				

#3 SWEET CONTINUED	LIKE IT	ACCEPTABLE	DON'T LIKE IT	DON'T KNOW
Ice cream				
Frozen yogurt				
Sorbets				
Prunes				
Fruit juices				
Muffins				
Hot cereal				
Pineapple				
Lychee (in syrup)				
Marmalade				
Yogurts (sweetened)				
Beets				
Teas (sweetened)				
Sweet bell peppers				
Sweet onions				
Corn				
Chutneys				
Ketchup				
Mangoes				
Parsnips				
Sweet potato / yam				
Nectarines				
Oranges				
Pears				
Plums				
Tangerines				
Peaches				
Carrots				
Bokchoy				
Tomato juice				
Rutabagas				

FOOD PREFERENCE SHEET

#3 SWEET CONTINUED	LIKE IT	ACCEPTABLE	DON'T LIKE IT	DON'T KNOW
Jicama				
Banana				
Figs				
Grapes				
Melon				
#4 BITTER	**LIKE IT**	**ACCEPTABLE**	**DON'T LIKE IT**	**DON'T KNOW**
Citrus zest				
Nuts				
Brussels sprouts				
Ryvita				
Broccoli				
Tomato paste				
Wheat kernels				
Rhubarb				
Chutneys				
Broad beans (fava), fresh				
Kiwi fruit				
Persimmons				
Collards				
Celeriac				
Eggplant				
Asparagus				
Cabbage				
Cauliflower				
Fennel				
Salad greens				
Green onions				
Cucumbers				
#5 UMAMI	**LIKE IT**	**ACCEPTABLE**	**DON'T LIKE IT**	**DON'T KNOW**
Cheese, Parmesan				
Fish sauce				

#5 UMAMI CONTINUED	LIKE IT	ACCEPTABLE	DON'T LIKE IT	DON'T KNOW
Dried lever seaweed				
Soy sauce				
Soy beans, fermented				
Onions				
Wakame seaweed				
Kelp seaweed				
Scallops				
Alaska king crab				
Blue crab				
Beets				
White shrimp				
Snow crab				
Apples				
Cheese, cheddar				
Eggs				
Chicken				
Beef				
Pork				
Cabbage				
Asparagus, green				
Mushrooms				
Salmon				
Avocado				
Cod				
Corn				
Green peas				
Shitake mushrooms				
Tomato				
Spinach				
Carrots				
Peppers				

FOOD PREFERENCE SHEET

#5 UMAMI CONTINUED	LIKE IT	ACCEPTABLE	DON'T LIKE IT	DON'T KNOW
Potatoes				
Grapes				
Kiwi				
Milk				

#6 VOLATILES	LIKE IT	ACCEPTABLE	DON'T LIKE IT	DON'T KNOW
Port				
Brandy				
Sherry				
Red wine				
Balsamic Vinegar				
White wine				
Soy sauce				
Vanilla, other essence				
Almond extract				

#7 PASSIVE	LIKE IT	ACCEPTABLE	DON'T LIKE IT	DON'T KNOW
Apples				
Apricots				
Avocados				
Bananas				
Raspberries				
Strawberries				
Blueberries				
Blackberries				
Cherries				
Dates				
Grapefruit				
Grape juice (and DA wines)				
Kiwi fruit				
Lemon				
Lime				
Mangoes				

#7 PASSIVE CONTINUED	LIKE IT	ACCEPTABLE	DON'T LIKE IT	DON'T KNOW
Nectarines				
Oranges and juices				
Papaya				
Peaches				
Pears				
Pineapple				
Tangerines				
Watermelon				
Melons (honeydew, etc.)				
Baked beans				
Beets				
Broccoli				
Cabbage				
Cauliflower				
Celeriac				
Celery				
Corn				
Fennel				
Green onions				
Ginger				
Marmalade				
Leeks				
Onions				
Parsnips				
Peas				
Peppers (sweet bell)				
Tomatoes				
Smoked salmon				
Parmesan cheese				
Nutritional yeast				
Olive oil (virgin)				

FOOD PREFERENCE SHEET

#7 PASSIVE CONTINUED	LIKE IT	ACCEPTABLE	DON'T LIKE IT	DON'T KNOW
Sesame seed (toasted)				
#8 PASSIVE	LIKE IT	ACCEPTABLE	DON'T LIKE IT	DON'T KNOW
Nut oils (avocado etc.)				
Bombay duck				
Sambal Oleck				
Thai fish sauce (NamPla)				
Anchovies				
Garlic				
Ginger (powdered)				
Ginger root				
Curry powder				
Allspice				
Clove				
Cumin				
Molasses				
Nutmeg				
Kimchee				
Oyster sauce				
Lemon grass				
Maple syrup				
Rosemary				
Citrus zests				
Fennel				
Anise				
Basil				
Cardamom				
Chili powder				
Oregano				
Tumeric				
Parmesan				
Peppercorns (fresh ground)				

#8 PASSIVE CONTINUED	LIKE IT	ACCEPTABLE	DON'T LIKE IT	DON'T KNOW
Saffron				
Canadian, bacon				
Mint				
Sage				
Thyme				
Worcestershire sauce				
Coconut essence				
Tarragon				
Vinegars, various				
Cocoa				
Ketchup				
Vanilla				
Caraway				
Cilantro				
Dill weed/seed				
Soy sauce				
Sour cream				
Buttermilk				
Bayleaf				
#9 OIL SACK/MALLIARD/ CARAMEL REACTIONS	LIKE IT	ACCEPTABLE	DON'T LIKE IT	DON'T KNOW
Garlic				
Ginger				
Green onions				
Citrus zest				
Leeks				
Cinnamon				
Clove				
Curry powder				
Garam Masala				
Fennel				

FOOD PREFERENCE SHEET

#9 OIL SACK/MALLIARD/ CARAMEL REACTIONS CONTINUED	LIKE IT	ACCEPTABLE	DON'T LIKE IT	DON'T KNOW
Chili powder				
Cumin				
Canadian bacon				
Tomatoes (esp. tomato paste)				
Ketchup				
Rosemary				
Saffron				
Sage				
Sweet corn				
Parsnips				
Chiles (hot-spicy)				
Coconut essence				
Bran muffins				
Bread				
Cookies				
Cakes/Pastries				
Peppers (sweet bell)				
Pumpkins (winter squash)				
Sweet potatoes				
Tomatillos				
Bagels				
Cornmeal				
Rutabagas				
Jasmine rice				
Cassava				
Potatoes				
Meats				
Poultry				
Eggs				

#10 RED	LIKE IT	ACCEPTABLE	DON'T LIKE IT	DON'T KNOW
Strawberries				
Peppers (sweet bell)				
Small peppers				
Peppers (red chili)				
Radish				
Tomatoes				
Crabapple				
Swiss chard stalks (raw)				
Red currants				
Paprika				
Cayenne				
Persimmons				
Cranberries (dried)				
Raspberries				
Cherries (fresh and dried)				
Kidney beans				

#11 ORANGE	LIKE IT	ACCEPTABLE	DON'T LIKE IT	DON'T KNOW
Oranges				
Marmalade				
Sweet potato				
Tangerines				
Carrots				
Peppers (sweet bell)				
Apricots				
Papaya				
Mango				
Pumpkin				
Acorn squash				
Hubbard squash				
Butternut squash				
Lentils ("red")				

FOOD PREFERENCE SHEET

#11 ORANGE	LIKE IT	ACCEPTABLE	DON'T LIKE IT	DON'T KNOW
Chickpeas (garbanzo beans)				
#12 PURPLE	**LIKE IT**	**ACCEPTABLE**	**DON'T LIKE IT**	**DON'T KNOW**
Beets				
Eggplant				
Blood orange				
Cherries (fresh & dried)				
Blueberries (deep)				
Blackberries (deep)				
Plums				
Grapes				
Peppers (sweet bell)				
Radish				
Carrots (purple)				
Potatoes				
Onions ("red")				
#13 YELLOW	**LIKE IT**	**ACCEPTABLE**	**DON'T LIKE IT**	**DON'T KNOW**
Peppers (sweet bell)				
Patti Pans summer squash				
Crookneck summer squash				
Whole eggs				
Eggbeaters				
Corn				
Tomatoes				
Pineapple				
Nectarines				
Peaches				
Cornmeal				
Parsnips (pale)				
Delicata squash				
Yellow fin potatoes (pale)				
Lentils				

#13 YELLOW CONTINUED	LIKE IT	ACCEPTABLE	DON'T LIKE IT	DON'T KNOW
Bananas (pale)				
Jerusalem artichokes				
#14 GREEN (LEAF)	**LIKE IT**	**ACCEPTABLE**	**DON'T LIKE IT**	**DON'T KNOW**
Swiss chard				
Collard				
Spinach				
Savory				
Beets (greens)				
Kale				
Mustard greens				
Bokchoy (tops)				
Romaine				
Arugula				
Watercress				
Pea vines				
Escarole				
Cabbage (drum head)				
Butterleaf				
Chinese (Napa)				
Curley endive				
Iceberg lettuce				
#15 GREEN	**LIKE IT**	**ACCEPTABLE**	**DON'T LIKE IT**	**DON'T KNOW**
Green beans				
Asparagus				
Soy beans (young)				
Peas, green				
Peas, snow				
Green onions				
Fennel tops				
Kiwi fruit				
Artichokes (globe)				

FOOD PREFERENCE SHEET

#15 GREEN CONTINUED	LIKE IT	ACCEPTABLE	DON'T LIKE IT	DON'T KNOW
Brussels sprouts				
Cherkin				
Capers				
Avocados				
Grapes (pale)				
Tomatillos (pale)				
Lima beans				
Celery (pale)				
Fava beans				
Cucumber				

#16 PINK	LIKE IT	ACCEPTABLE	DON'T LIKE IT	DON'T KNOW
Salmon				
Shrimp, flesh				
Cherries				
Lobster, flesh				
Crab, flesh				
Arctic char				
Watermelon				
Radish				
Swiss chard stalks				
Grapefruit				
Pickled ginger				
Rhubarb				

#17 BROWN & DEEPER COLORS	LIKE IT	ACCEPTABLE	DON'T LIKE IT	DON'T KNOW
Beans, black				
Chocolate				
Dates				
Coffee, instant				
Raisins				
Cocoa				
Wild rice				

#17 BROWN & DEEPER COLORS CONTINUED	LIKE IT	ACCEPTABLE	DON'T LIKE IT	DON'T KNOW
Meats, surface cooked				
Nuts, various				
Balsamic vinegar				
Garam masala				
Soy sauce				
Tomato paste (malliard)				
Beans, various				
Bread				
Muffins				
Cookies				
Doughnuts				
Pastry				
Wheat kernels				
Sultanas				
Bulgur				
Brown rice (pale)				

#18 WHITE/CREAM	LIKE IT	ACCEPTABLE	DON'T LIKE IT	DON'T KNOW
Potato				
Bagel (inside)				
Egg white				
Scallops				
Bokchoy (stalks)				
Vanilla ice cream				
Vanilla iced yogurt				
Yogurt				
Cream				
Icing sugar				
Fish (some)				
Fennel				
Milks				

FOOD PREFERENCE SHEET

#18 WHITE/CREAM CONTINUED	LIKE IT	ACCEPTABLE	DON'T LIKE IT	DON'T KNOW
Daikon (radish)				
Water chestnut				
Soy				
Rice				
Pasta				
Noodles				
Soy beans (dried)				
Endive (chicory)				
Udon				
Yam				
Tofu				
Lychee				
Butterbeans				
Navy beans				
Celeriac				
Jicama				
Onions				
Eggplant (inside)				
Barley				
Couscous				
Cassava				
White asparagus				
Turnips				
Yam				
Quinoa				
Chicken				
Apple (inside)				
Oatmeal (darker)				
Bamboo shoots				
Gnocchi				
Turkey				

#18 WHITE/CREAM CONTINUED	LIKE IT	ACCEPTABLE	DON'T LIKE IT	DON'T KNOW
Popcorn				
Bananas				
Evaporated skim milk				
Rutabagas (deep cream)				
Taro				

#19 SPICY	LIKE IT	ACCEPTABLE	DON'T LIKE IT	DON'T KNOW
Habanero peppers (Scotch Bonnet)				
Datil pepper				
Wasabi (green mustard)				
Jalapeno pepper				
Horseradish				
White peppercorn				
Black peppercorn				
Hot sauces, various				
Tabasco				
Mustards, various				
Anaheim pepper				
Radish				
Arugula (rocket)				

#20 MOUTH ROUND FULLNESS (MRF)	LIKE IT	ACCEPTABLE	DON'T LIKE IT	DON'T KNOW
Custards				
Flan (molded custards)				
Butter				
Eggs				
Margarine, various				
Cream				
Chocolate				
Smoothies				
Bananas				

FOOD PREFERENCE SHEET

#20 MOUTH ROUND FULLNESS (MRF) CONTINUED	LIKE IT	ACCEPTABLE	DON'T LIKE IT	DON'T KNOW
Nut butters				
Avocado				
Oatmeal				
Bagel				
Pear				
Scallops				
Arrowroot				
Root vegetables as "velvet" (purees)				
Peas and corn as "velvet" (purees)				
Yogurt cheese				
Ice cream				
Gelatin (Agar)				
Yogurt				
Cheese				
Hummus				
Spinach as saag (Indian cooking)				
Cornstarch				
Potato starch				
Pasta				
Cornmeal (polenta)				
Milk				
Cassava (Manioc)				

INDEX OF SPECIAL HELPS

INDEX OF RECIPES